The healing power of
COLOUR

Examines what colour does to us, how it can be used in
magic and dream interpretation, and how we can use it to
improve our behaviour and our health.

The healing power of
COLOUR

How to use colour to improve your mental, physical
and spiritual well-being

by

Betty Wood

THE AQUARIAN PRESS
Wellingborough, Northamptonshire

First published 1984
Second Impression 1985
Third Impression 1986

British Library Cataloguing in Publication Data

Wood, Betty
   The Healing power of colour.
   1. Color — Physiological effect
   2. Color — Therapeutic use
   I. Title
   613'.1   QP82.2.L5

   ISBN 0-85030-384-2

*The Aquarian Press is part of the
Thorsons Publishing Group*

Printed and bound in Great Britain

Contents

Introduction

In a book about colour and colour healing it is important to understand that we do not have to visually perceive colour for it to have some effect on us. Colour on its own and in the form of light continuously affects those subtler senses and autonomous processes that ultimately play such a significant part in our lives.

Colour-blind people, for instance, may be totally unable to see colours such as red and green and at worst may only see a grey world. The totally blind from birth may only have the haziest idea of what we mean by colour. However, Professor Harold Wohlfarth, a photobiologist at the University of Alberta and President of the German Academy of Color Science, believes that colour certainly has a physiological effect. In an experiment he found that light had an 'identical' influence on the blood-pressure and pulse of two blind children as on seven sighted children. He contends that light colours cause reactions in one or more of the brain's neurotransmitters. But it also seems that in certain cases it can affect other parts of the body, if recent experiments in China and Russia are anything to go by. It is claimed in these instances that a number of people have been able to see colours, and read, with different parts of their bodies other than the eyes.

Each of us sees colour in a slightly different way, although we might call it by the same name. Even so, two people may disagree as to whether a colour is, say, blue or lilac. Some languages have no words for complex colours and, like children and early man, find the primary colours the most attractive and the easiest to describe and remember.

'Let there be light' is the primal cry of many creation myths, for without the action of the 'Sun God' life would never have manifested as it did. Of course as we know, light has a very important effect on all growing things through the process of photosynthesis, and on all living creatures including the human, on whose reproductive processes it has a significant effect. In the stronger form of sunlight it promotes the formation of vitamins in the body, especially vitamin C, and in some instances vitamin *deficiency* — as can happen after over-exposure to certain types of fluorescent lighting. Light striking the retina appears to influence the pineal gland's synthesis of melatonin, a hormone that helps determine the body's output of serotonin, a neurotransmitter. Professor Wohlfarth is at present conducting experiments along these lines in four schools and some very interesting results are appearing. Also, according to Alexander Schauss, director of the American Institute for Biosocial Research, the electro-magnetic energy of colour affects the pituitary and pineal glands, and the hypothalamus, all of which have a profound influence on the bodily system. While it is still a matter of controversy amongst scientists and psychologists, they all have to agree that certainly the sections of the electro-magnetic spectrum which we cannot see, such as X-rays, microwaves and ultraviolet rays, do definitely affect the physical body, so it does not seem impossible that the section of the spectrum that we can actually see can also affect us in various ways.

Life would be somewhat flavourless without the stimulation of colour — how we use it can tell us a lot about ourselves and may tell other people even more! If we are unwise in our colour schemes we may give quite the wrong impression to others, or we may be so drab as to slip by unnoticed and wonder why we never make an impact! Colour, therefore, affects the whole of our lives — in our homes, our places of work and play, our dress, and behaviour. Further in the book we shall perhaps gain insight as to why we choose certain colours in preference to others and how, by careful use of colour, we can change the mood of a room or even the attitude of another person towards us.

Psychologists disagree between themselves as to the significance of colour in the human personality but, as in the Lüscher Test, of which more later, there seems to be a correlation between colour and personality. While much of this may be due to cultural influences and upbringing, if we go back to prehistoric days we can see how important colour was to early man and how it has evolved. But human intuition is a very useful guide also and in the long term will probably prove more reliable than a dozen psychological personality tests.

Colour has texture, taste and feel — some people even hear it as a corresponding musical note: slow, heavy music conjures up blues and darker colours while a rapid tempo is at the red end of the spectrum; high-pitched tones bring light colours to the mind and low-pitched, dark colours. Psychologists think this is probably based on inherited traits but have no really satisfactory explanation. To some people, every day of the week is a different colour, which never changes throughout their lives. Numbers are different colours, and names evoke different colours — all Michaels are say, green, and all Elizabeths, blue.

We also carry around with us our own personal electrical field known as the 'aura'. This is somewhat similar to the Earth's aurora, with positive north at the head and negative south at the feet. The most brilliant display is usually around the head and this can be seen to some degree by most people after a little practice of knowing what to look for. This is an important indicator of health and mood and state of mind, and can be rapidly assessed by someone particularly gifted in this way. For us lesser mortals, however, if we can only partially see or even not see the aura at all, there is no cause for dismay — unless particularly unaware, most of us can sense an aura and in any case react automatically as an attractive or hostile auric field approaches us.

In short, we are subtly, and sometimes dramatically, influenced by colour all the time. A bright orange or red poster comes forward to grab us — while the gentler colours of blue and green appear to draw back and lead us on. Advertisers catch the eye by careful arrangement of shapes and colours, much as the flower attracts the bee.

Finally, how we see and use colour in all its varied shades, tones and hues may be but a reflection of our inner memories. Some of the most beautiful examples of colour — an opalescent dawn of gold and rose, the luminous blue of an evening sky, sunlight through stained glass windows or a rainbow spanning the heavens, may well bring to our minds a far away remembrance of some other realm, where light and colour weave patterns we can only guess at. Our dreams and meditations bring back a glimpse of these and, used wisely in our quest for healing and wholeness, they can only have a beneficial and harmonizing effect.

1.
Colour In Our Past

If we search back in time in an endeavour to trace the evolution of colour awareness and sensitivity, to a great extent we can only speculate. Such speculation is however often validated by discoveries in archaeology and anthropology. Our earliest known ancestors, Cro-Magnon Man and Neanderthal Man, have only left small traces of their existence — stone tools, bone implements, fragments of human skeleton and occasional burial places. The most exciting finds have been the cave paintings, executed with superb craftsmanship and coloured with natural materials — various pigments to which prehistoric man had fairly easy access.

Of these early attempts at colouring, the most obvious conclusion is that man looked around him at his environment and the creatures and plants that flourished in abundance; at the sky, the sun and moon, the rivers and the sea. And at himself. He saw the colours of the earth, of fire and blood and water, fur and feathers in all their great variety, and brightly-hued reptiles and insects. He found materials to hand such as red ochre, an oxidized earth that ranges in colour from yellow to purple, also known as bloodstone or haematite. Neanderthal skeletal remains have been found lying in a bed of red ochre, or sometimes the bones were painted with it, a practice still carried on today for instance, by Bushmen in Australia.

This pigment would not be regarded simply as a means of decoration but as very special material symbolic of various sacred powers and principles needing to be invoked for aid and protection. In Africa stone tools dating back to prehistoric times have been found adjacent to old mine workings dating back some 50,000 years. Archaeologists have been reluctant to admit that these mines were worked by prehistoric man, as he was not known to have discovered the use of metal ore. Instead they

have overlooked the fact that he may have been mining for pigment instead. Now, in a recent book by Lyall Watson, *Lightning
Bird*, appears a most convincing argument that early man did in
fact mine for pigment in much the same way as do present-day
Africans.

Lightning Bird is the true story of a young man, Adrian
Boshier, who early in life determined to go to Africa and ex-
plore it on foot. He became a legend in his time not only for his
snake-handling abilities but also for his knowledge and experience of native culture. A priestess-diviner, Rrasebe, took
him under her wing and taught him many of her secrets. One
day she took him to some caves and told him how she
remembered her father working with his paints. He would
grind white stone, charcoal and red earth and mix them with
water and other liquids. Having obtained the desired result, he
would then paint traditional designs and patterns on the rocks.
'Throughout Africa,' says Lyall Watson, 'colour plays an important role in symbolism, particularly that related to
medicine.' As a result of this knowledge and the actual
discovery of prehistoric tools in Swaziland, Adrian Boshier interested a well-known paleontologist, Professor Dart, who gave
him advice and help. It seems likely from their joint research,
and in comparison with tools Professor Dart had found in Zam-
bia, that shamanistic priests and diviners still use similar tools
and methods of extraction for pigments such as crystals of
manganese dioxide and pyrolusite (also very much valued in
Ancient Egypt) as their forefathers did thousands of years
before.

In Africa important colours are black, red and white. Not too
surprisingly, black is the colour of night, death, excrement, and
illness, while white is daylight, life, food, and good health. Red
indicates a transformation — the red of sunrise is a move
towards health and the red of sunset a decline into disease.
However, for the Maasai, black is a very important colour with
many positive aspects — it symbolizes the colour of
thunderclouds, for example — a much desired sight in the dry
season.

What applies to peoples in Africa could also well apply to
similar cultures in other parts of the world — Europe, Asia and
the Americas. One of the first colours most likely to have made
a great impact on man was red — the colour of blood and fire.
Blood was the source of mysterious power, the life force,

irreplaceable and mystical, the mainstream of life. A blood sacrifice was the greatest thing Man could give to his gods — his, or preferably something or someone's very life energy. We who consider ourselves civilized can hardly imagine now the effect of such a ceremony upon a group of people whose lives and beliefs were so very basic, although to some extent the blood sacrifice still goes on in some parts of the world. We may even have our modern equivalent in the daily slaughter on the roads. Fire also, its association with the sun, its warmth and protection so essential, its destructive power and mystery, made it one of the most potent sacred symbols.

Black, with its negative associations, would also be a very special colour, signifying all those fearful, dark and hidden forces of nature and the unknown from which early man had to protect himself. Its opposite, white, represented the lighter, happier, positive qualities that made life enjoyable. It does not take too much imagination to connect yellow with the sun and thus symbolize another form of life. Gradually, no doubt, more colours became available from minerals, seeds, plants and insects. Lapis lazuli, turquoise and various gem stones possibly gave painters ideas for coloration so that by the time of the earliest civilizations there was a wide range of materials available for painting and personal decoration. Colour was absolutely essential for its protective and magical qualities — it would drive off evil spirits and encourage good ones to help and protect. The shamans or priests of the tribe would probably be responsible for rock and cave paintings and it would be their choice of colours and pigments that set the scene for everyone else. Shamanism is the oldest known religion on earth and most likely the precursor of all later cults, being derived from man's deepest roots and oldest, most basic beliefs and feelings. Early man, and most peoples living close to nature, were and still are highly sensitive to their natural environment and in their dreams and visions would perceive the 'gods' and the various colours associated with them. There has been some talk of various rock paintings in Africa depicting 'spacemen' but it seems much more realistic to consider that these strange figures, with 'globes' around their heads and various ritualistic implements in their hands, are denizens of the dream world and part of a remarkably consistent pattern experienced by native 'seers' around the world, the archetypes of mankind's inner life and of the great life principles at work in the universe.

Dr R.M. Bucke, author of *Cosmic Consciousness*, a 'classic' well worth reading on many counts, has put forward an interesting theory regarding the evolution of the colour sense in mankind. He takes the analogy of childhood development and compares this to the gradual evolution of early man. In the child, he maintains, memory appears a few days after birth, then after a few weeks simple consciousness and curiosity develop; then, at a few years , use of tools, and finally self-consciousness, followed shortly by awareness of colour and fragrance. No doubt this varies with individual children and may likewise vary with individual races.

Dr Bucke quotes an early researcher, Lazarus Geiger (1880), who pointed out that it could be proved by examination of language that as late in the life of the race as the ancient Aryans, perhaps not more than 15 or 20,000 years ago, man was only conscious of, and only perceived, one colour. That is to say he did not distinguish between blue sky and green trees and grass, or brown or grey earth. All these colours might be described by the one word 'black'. Adolphe Pictet (1877), another researcher, reported that he found no names of colours in primitive Indo-European speech. Max Mueller (1887) a language researcher, found no Sanskrit root whose meaning has any reference to colour.

At a later period when the main part of the *Rig Veda* (early Sanskrit writings) was composed, red, yellow and black were recognized as three separate colours; still later white was added to the list and then eventually green, but through the *Rig Veda*, the Zend Avesta, the Homeric poems with their 'wine-dark' sea[1] and the Bible, claims Dr Bucke, the colour of the sky is not once mentioned. He therefore concludes that blue was not recognized. However, although this is an intriguing idea it is not altogether convincing, especially from the point of view of blue not being recognised. For instance in the Bible blue is mentioned many times — Ezekiel 23.6 mentions 'horsemen clothed with blue, captains and rulers' and 'blue and purple from the Isles of Elishah'. Apart from Joseph's coat of many colours, in Exodus 25.4 offerings are described as 'blue and purple, and scarlet...and gold'. In Esther 1.6 'white, green and blue hangings' and 'royal apparel of blue and white' are described. Ezekiel likens God unto a rainbow: 'As the appearance of the bow that is in the cloud in the day of rain, so was the appearance of the brightness round about.' And on another occasion 'God' was seen standing on 'As it were a paved work of sapphire stone, and as it were the very heaven for clearness.' So it seems rather unlikely that in biblical days people were unable to see or describe the colour blue. Green also appears many times — 'green pastures' in Psalm 23.2, 'green herbs' in Genesis, while Jacob (Gen.30.7) 'took him rods of green poplar'. Most other colours also have extensive mention.

Basically however we come back to red, black, white and yellow as the earliest colours. When Dr Leonard Woolley excavated the ziggurat at Ur, one of the oldest buildings in the world, he found that it was built in four stages, the lowest being black and the uppermost red. Pursuing his theory, Dr Bucke states that the English word 'blue' and the German 'blau' are said to descend from a word that meant black, also that the Chinese hi-u-an which now means sky blue, formerly meant black. Nil, which in Persian and Arabic means blue, is derived from the name Nile, which meant Black River, of which the Latin Niger is a form. Dr Bucke considered that under the designation 'red' were included white, yellow and all intermediate tints; while under 'black' were included all shades of blue and green.

There is a rapid decrease in the energy of light waves as we pass along the spectrum from red to violet, and if as Dr Bucke suggests, the eye evolved according to the power of a light wave to excite vision, it would seem natural that red, having energy rays several thousand times as great as blue and violet, would be the first colour perceived, followed by yellow, then green, and so on to violet. He cites various studies undertaken by researchers to determine the incidence of colour-blindness. It seems that four per cent of European males suffer from it to some extent, and 0.25 per cent of females, the incidence being slightly lower for Chinese males at three per cent. However, that among Japanese was much less and it might be surmised, rightly or wrongly, that as a race their colour sense evolved at a very early date. Certainly they are one of the most artistic and colour-aware of the world's peoples.

Dr Bucke considered colour-blindness to be a modern phenomenon of possible atavistic origin and not properly belonging to this age. It is an intriguing thought that perhaps in the far distant future mankind will acquire an extended colour range, maybe even comparable to that of the bee.

Once the great civilizations began to develop, naturally colour with its important magical qualities was extensively used. One likes to think also that maybe by then, if not before, *homo sapiens* had also developed a sense of beauty and did not regard colour simply as a practical necessity. As far as orthodox archaeology tells us, the Mesopotamians (Chaldeans) are perhaps the earliest recorded 'civilizations' as such, living in cities and organizing themselves to quite a degree of sophistication. Tradition has it that the Chaldeans were the ancient Magi—masters of magic and astrology, who dedicated their temples to planetary gods of the heavens. James Fergusson in his *History of Architecture in All Countries* (1893), tells us that they decorated these temples in the appropriate colours depending on which god had his abode there. Herodotus refers to what seems to be the great temple of Nebuchadnezzar at Barsippa, which was 272 feet square at its base. It rose in seven stages, each one being set back away from a central point. It was found that this temple was dedicated to the seven planets and decorated with the colours of each. Thus the lower stage was black, the colour of Saturn; the next, orange for Jupiter; the third, red for Mars; the fourth yellow for the sun; and the fifth and sixth, green and blue respectively for Venus and Mercury, and the upper probably white for the Moon, whose place in the Chaldean system would be extremely important. Present day astrologers differ amongst themselves somewhat as to planetary colours, as will be seen later.

Next came the Egyptians. Their temples, tombs and presumably their homes were decorated inside and out with bright, clear colours of black, red, yellow, green, blue and purple. 'Colour' meant the same as substance,[2] of which colour was an important part. If one said of the gods that one 'could not know their colour' it meant that one could not know their substance, their essence. Emotional qualities were attributed to certain colours — red therefore being aggressive and suggesting danger, but also life-giving. It would be placed alongside blue, which is subdued and yet flowing out to infinity. The gods and goddesses had their special colours denoting their various qualities. Osiris, for instance, was sometimes referred to as 'the great green' and was often painted green because of his associations with fertility, resurrection and death. He was also known as 'the Black One' no doubt due to his association with the Underworld. Black, as in earlier cultures, was a reference to death and the netherworld but also of rebirth and resurrection. Bread made from white grain and beer from red were food and drink in the netherworld. In other instances the two colours became opposites as in the case of hippopotami where the 'red' male animal and the 'white' female were regarded as hostile and helpful respectively. The Egyptians not only decorated their buildings and sculptures but also themselves, using say red paint and jewellery for a particular festival, probably much the same as present-day Hindus scatter around various coloured substances, particularly red and yellow, at religious festivals. While Egyptian art remained stylized for the most part over the several thousand years of their culture, there were periods when the country was in a state of instability and art suffered accordingly. They have nevertheless bequeathed to us a legacy which still influences our colour utilization today — most notably perhaps in religious ceremonial clothes, which are often scarlet. Red often symbolized life and victory and red and white together (as in our own St George's flag) expressed wholeness and perfection. The White Crown of Upper Egypt and the Red Crown of Lower Egypt were worn together to symbolize the unity and balance of the whole country.

Sometimes red took on a more negative aspect as it was also the colour of Set, god of the desert and of the typhoon, the negative force in Egyptian mythology. Set was thought to have red eyes and red hair (the colour of the desert) and thus a person 'with a red heart' was considered to be in a rage, 'to redden' meant the same as 'to die'. There was a red lake of fire in the Underworld in which the damned were punished — another legacy for us! 'To do red things' meant to do evil, while to 'do green things' meant the opposite.

White became expressive of earthly omnipotence, a way of symbolizing sacred things, and was the colour of purity and sanctity. Being also the colour of joy, a cheerful person was referred to as 'white'. Gold symbolized the Sun and all its various attributes, and would be the natural choice for the colour for the god Ra. The god Amun was coloured blue because of his cosmic associations.

Early Egyptian and Greek temple decorations may have appeared rather garish to our eyes, accustomed as we are to the mellow gold-beige of the present-day ruins. But many examples of Egyptian decoration are still around for all to see, and it takes no great stretch of imagination to apply this also to the Greek and Roman temples of later date. As with the Egyptians, Greek marble statues would often be highly coloured, with red lips, and eyes decorated in yellow, green and blue, often with eyelashes as well. Particularly impressive are those statues with eyes made of precious stones, which must have been most awe-inspiring when first seen gleaming out of the darkness of a tomb, shining like the eyes of a cat. Some find it rather painful to consider that the exterior of the Parthenon, for instance, was similarly embellished with bright colours of red, blue, yellow, gold and black decorating the cornices, friezes and columns. The Romans as usual followed suit, the Gods determining the colour choice. Purple, or a magenta colour, would be reserved for the Emperor in his role as the personification of Jupiter. Although unfortunate for the inhabitants, it is our gain that Pompeii and Herculaneum were preserved under volcanic ash sufficiently for us to see the wonderful paintings and artwork of that time. Likewise in the palace of Minos in Crete, dating back to 1600 B.C. and before, many restorations can be seen of the original wall paintings and decorations in red, yellow, blue, brown and black, with red and black the predominant colours.

Another ancient people to whom colour was very significant were the Chinese. In fact their various dynasties were represented by colours — brown for the Sun, green for Ming, yellow for Ch'ing. Predictably enough, the emperor wore blue when worshipping sky deities, and yellow for earth. The Chinese had five primary colours — red, yellow, black, white and green, which in turn corresponded to the five elements — fire, metal, wood, earth and water, to the five happinesses, the five virtues, the five vices, and the five precepts of faith. Their subsequent discovery of jade in all its varied and delicate shades no doubt enlarged their colour sense immensely. We seem to think we are today the only people with regard to the beauty of nature and the value of wild creatures, but one has only to look at the accurate and expressive drawings of animals, birds and all other creatures as portrayed by the artists of these early cultures to see that although portraying all of nature with a true and unsentimental eye, they drew and painted, one might say, from the heart.

Returning to China for a moment, red, as in almost every other culture was regarded as the positive, masculine essence, and yellow as the earthly and feminine principle. Buildings were often painted red, symbolic of the south, sun and happiness, with yellow roofs symbolic of the earth. When a home was built, red firecrackers were exploded and a piece of red cloth suspended to promote happiness and well-being. Green pine branches were placed on top of the scaffolding to deceive wandering evil spirits into thinking they were passing over a forest. Red and yellow are the marriage hues for the Orient in general, Egypt, Russia and the Balkans. It is not surprising that red in China is regarded as the luckiest of colours, representing the sun and the phoenix bird. Orange also represents love and happiness, while blue denoted the Azure Dragon of the East, the heavens, clouds and the spring.

While it would be tedious to enumerate colours as used by every culture since these early days, it might be useful to see the correspondences between various widespread areas of the world. Red is almost universally regarded as the most positive, creative and life-giving colour. It does however, as we have seen, have its negative side. In Celtic mythology red meant disaster and is symbolic of martyrdom, cruelty and zeal in the Christian church.

Black is associated with primordial darkness and everything negative. It also signifies time and is associated with the dark aspect of the Great Mother, especially as the Hindu goddess Kali, who is Kala, time, and with black virgins. Black or blue-black is the colour of chaos, of storm clouds. In Christian tradition it symbolizes the Prince of Darkness, hell, death etc. and spiritual darkness, the unconscious, but also in Hebraic Qabalistic tradition, mercy and understanding. But the general concensus of opinion seems to incline to the idea of black as a negative, frightening colour.

White, naturally enough, usually represents the opposite. Whilst having associations of both life and death, it usually stands for wholeness, purity and innocence and is a most sacred colour. Used by the Chinese and sometimes the Romans for mourning, it nevertheless has associations of spiritual authority. Buddhists regard it as the colour of self-mastery while the ancient Egyptians, who wore a lot of it, considered white and green as symbolic of joy. White and of course silver also relate to the Moon and the unconscious, feminine side of mankind.

Yellow nearly everywhere stands for the Sun, along with gold, and signifies divine power, enlightenment and immortality. In Hinduism gold is life, truth, light, immortality, the seed and the sign of Agni (the Hindu god of fire). The

Buddhists regard it as the colour of renunciation, desirelessness and humility and often wear ochre robes which it is believed were adopted because they were originally worn by condemned criminals and outcasts. It is a colour öf mostly happy associations — of sun and brightness, light and life. But like other colours it has its negative side and dark yellow can signify treachery, faithlessness and betrayal.

Next, one would think, comes blue and all its associations of sky and water. Most cultures connect it with truth, revelation, wisdom, loyalty, fertility, constancy and chastity. Blue is the colour of the great deeps, the feminine principle, the Great Mother. In the West the blue cloak of the Mother Goddess is a vastly protective and comforting symbol, evocative of peace, compassion and healing. We even incorporate a little bit of it in our 'something borrowed, something blue' for the bride. Blue is a colour that one can sink into, a view with which most ancients might agree. It is the colour of infinity and infinite peace, the wisdom of Dharma-Dhatu in Buddhist thought. In Celtic mythology blue denoted the bard or poet, the raincloak of Indra, the war and fertility god of the Hindus. For Qabalists it is the colour of mercy. Everyone seems to love blue, although at times it can denote coolness and remoteness.

Along comes green, with its associations of nature in all its aspects, the cycle of birth and death. In Buddhist ideology vernal green denotes everything pertaining to life, while pale green signifies death. In Christian thought also, vernal green denotes immortality, hope, and the growth of the Holy Spirit in Man, triumph over death, and the annual resurrection of spring after winter, while similarly pale green signifies Satan, evil and death. Possibly the most noteworthly quality of green is that of transformation, life and death, abundance on one hand and unripeness and immaturity, and even decay, on the other. It has soothing and harmonizing qualities and neutralizes the pushiness and energy of red. In Qabalism green stands for victory and it is also the sacred colour of Islam. Strangely enough in the West it is often regarded as unlucky because of its links with 'the Little People'. It is their colour and it might upset them to see humans wearing it. Or perhaps the Church frowned on its associations with fertility, being only too aware of the Call of Pan which can lure your soul away, never to be redeemed!

Brown, an earthly colour and one of the oldest, is usually

symbolic of the Earth and although frequently used in paintings, does not seem to have been particularly sacred. It can denote death to the world and negation of personality, as when used by some religious orders, as is black, also it can symbolize penitence and a renunciation of earthly things.

Violet and purple probably came a little later on the scene and the discovery of the Murex shellfish no doubt gave a wonderful boost to the Phoenician economy. From this they acquired the dye for their 'Tyrrhenian purple' so much in demand for royalty and for ceremonial robes. For the Aztec and Inca cultures it stands for majesty and sovereignty, while in the West it is the colour of Jupiter, and religious devotion. It usually seems connected with spiritual values and was reserved for certain privileged persons. Today it is still used for special occasions, being a rather 'heavy' colour to wear and needing a strong personality or grand occasion to carry it off successfully. Lesser shades of violet and lilac often have spiritual connotations.

The above were the main colours used but of course orange, grey, pink, and all their variations were also used. Gold and silver were inevitably the sun and the moon, the one rich and warm and the other cool and delicate. In Qabalism grey represents wisdom, and orange, splendour. Many ancient peoples gave specific colours to the four corners of the earth but these vary from place to place between such widely diverse cultures as Old Irish, Mayan and North American Indians. As used in Navaho sand paintings today, white represents the universal cosmic energy and black is the great void from which all comes; red is life and energy; yellow, the sun; and blue, spirituality.

From these early days colour awareness took off with a splendour which has rarely been matched since. The Byzantines revelled in the lavish use of colour of a richness and brilliance which may cause some to prefer the simplicity of earlier times. And then came the Renaissance, its painting and sculpture lighting up the whole of the Middle Ages as if after a period of spiritual darkness all the candles in the world had been lit. Many secrets of colour have been lost as master painters, glassblowers and stained glass artists guarded their recipes so carefully that no-one was able to repeat them. A barrister, Charles Winston (1847) managed to rediscover some of the medieval constituents of coloured glass.[3] He and Dr Medlock of the Royal College of Chemistry found, for example, that the most beautiful blue was obtained not from lapis lazuli, as had been previously thought, but from cobalt. Kazakh (USSR) scientists have likewise recently rediscovered the formula for the glazing used to decorate medieval architectural monuments after studying the multi-coloured patterns of the fourteenth century artist, Ahmad Yasavi. They established that the old mural painters used sand and clay as basic materials, with other necessary components obtained from the ashes of 'sarychob' roots.

Stained glass in England owes much of its wonderful brilliance to the various recipes used by generations of craftsmen but it also owes a great deal to our climate with its greyer light, which shows stained glass to much greater advantage than does the brilliant sunshine of the Mediterranean and Far East. Coloured glass was regarded as particularly precious from early monastic days. Theophilus, a German monk writing in the first half of the twelfth century, in his treatise *On Divers Arts* goes into considerable detail about the making of windows, but carefully leaves out chapters which give precise instructions for the colouring of glass with copper, lead and salt. This would be one of the secret recipes so jealously guarded. June Osborne, author of *Stained Glass in England*, writes that 'In religious terms, light was a symbol of vital importance, used to describe the quality of spirit itself.' And stained glass, while much more expensive than plain 'could be used to fill the congregation with a sense of mystery and vision and also had the function of glorifying God for his own sake.' 'Like an intelligent enquirer,' wrote Theophilus. 'I have laboured to inform myself, by all methods, what invention of art and vitality of colour may beautify a structure and not repel the light of day and the rays of the sun.' Specimens of coloured glass have been found in Saxon monastic buildings of the seventh or eighth century and there is a remarkable range of colour, considering the possibly rather limited range of materials available. Several shades of red, turquoise, viridian, eau-de-nil, four different shades of yellow, violet and a very pale violet, and white glass streaked with purple, are among the colours used. Francis Wilson Oliphant (1855) a glass-painter among other things, says 'the power of glass... to convey colour is quite unique; no kind of painting can at all come up to it. Glass is... a luminous material, full of points which catch the light like the facets of a diamond.'

Many of the great painters have also striven after this quality of luminosity, particularly for religious paintings, and again there have been many secret recipes, some of which have been lost and some rediscovered. Glass lustre artifacts also reflect this quality and it is obviously something integral in the human being that requires this reminder of, as mentioned in the Introduction, other realities than the ordinary, everyday appearance of things. Socrates in the *Phaedo*, in describing the 'real earth' says of it that 'the colours which we know are only limited samples, like the paints which artists use; but there the whole earth is made up of such colours, and others far brighter and purer still... even these very hollows in the earth, full of water and air, assume a kind of colour as they gleam amid the different hues around them, so that there appears to be one continuous surface of varied colours.' Gems also have this peculiar quality of luminesence, a hidden fire in their depths, which again stirs some long-forgotten memory. Ancient literature is full of such remarks as '... has the appearance of a sapphire' or '... was the colour of amber', or again '...a rainbow round the throne, in sight like unto an emerald.' (Revelations). The description of the New Jerusalem includes walls of jasper, garnished with all manner of precious stones, and of course we all know of the pearly gates!

Josephus, the Jewish historian in the first century AD associated white with earth, red with fire, purple with water, and yellow with air. However fifteen centuries later Leonardo da Vinci stated his colour preferences as 'white for the representative of light, without which no colour can be seen; yellow for the earth; green for water; blue for air; red for fire; and black for total darkness.' Some of these colours are still included in astrological tradition, as with yellow for Mercury and air, and things intellectual; red for Mars, fire and energy.

So fashions and preferences do tend to change and evolve — in one era nobles, warriors, middleclass and peasants tend to wear distinguishing colours, as in early Aryan cultures, or at other times certain colours are reserved for specific trades and professions, as today in law, religion and the armed forces; faculties at universities and colleges have their special colours; children at school have their team colours; and in many sports colours are extremely important, not only in order that contestants may identify one another, but that the audience may also identify them. All over the world colours of symbolic significance have been woven into tapestries and beadwork, painted on icons, walls, pottery and stonework, incorporated into inlay work and stained glass, glass vessels and jewellery, not only for ornamentation and visual enjoyment, but for the practice of sympathetic and protective magic in all its aspects, and ultimately and simply for the glory of God.

To return to the Chaldeans for a moment, their traditions have no doubt influenced later generations down to present day, particularly those engaged in magic and astrology. Qabalism is one example where the use of colour is essential to 'set the scene' for magical working. Other esoteric traditions in the West also use colours for their rituals and workings, as can be seen from the teachings of such organizations as The Order of the Golden Dawn, which has given rise to many similar and breakaway movements. For example, if one wishes to conjure up the power of the Sun God in his guise as Apollo, or Ra or whatever, gold and yellow would be the predominant colours to use — altar cloths, flowers, ritual implements, clothing, ornaments and so on, would all repeat the theme of gold and yellow. Likewise with the Moon, where silver, white and perhaps touches of green or violet would be essential. All the planetary 'gods' have their special colours, although these do vary a little between different esoteric and astrological traditions. Mostly however, colours tend to be grouped as follows:

Sun — gold, bright yellow — with its astrological sign Leo being assigned red, gold and sometimes yellow-green.
Moon — silver, white and emerald green — and often darker green and grey in smoky hues for its astrological subject Cancer.
Mars — red, of course, crimson, scarlet and similar shades — while Aries, its zodiacal subject, often has red and white as its colours. The old barber-surgeon's pole — a Martian occupation if ever there was one, is of course striped red and white — which may therefore not just be an allusion to blood and bandages. Mars is also the ruler of Scorpio and here the darker shades of red apply.
Venus — ruler again of two astrological signs, Taurus and Libra, all three sharing the colours of blue, blue-green and turquoise.

Mercury — another somewhat volatile ruler of two signs, is usually associated with yellow or orange, while some opinions also add lilac and off white. Gemini and Virgo, his subjects, share these colours.

Jupiter — the royal planet — purple, of course, sometimes violet or russet reds, shared by its subject Sagittarius.

Saturn — with reputedly sober Capricorn, is assigned olive green and grey, sometimes dark greens and black.

Uranus — and Aquarius, two somewhat erratic areas of the zodiac, favour electric blue, pale greens or citrine, always light colours.

Neptune — the mystical planet happiest in Pisces, has been assigned several colours — dark blue, indigo, greys, green — but all of a filmy nature. Some traditions use pink or coral.

Pluto — the enigma not yet assigned to any particular area and therefore still a bit undecided. Yellow, pale green or navy blue have been suggested, so you'll have to use your own feelings as a guide to this one.

Earth — our own planet is often assigned lavender blue or white.

So if you are wanting to work your own rituals, not only are there many books giving guidelines and colour correspondences in this respect, but you can use your own intuition. After studying the qualities of the 'god' or 'cosmic principle' which you wish to invoke, set up your own colour scheme for the 'working' which most appeals to you, both aesthetically and intellectually, and which 'feels right'. You may find some helpful ideas in later chapters.

References

1. There is some controversy over the phrase 'wine-dark sea'. Two Canadian scientists claim that the explanation lies in Greek water, which is strongly alkaline and when added to wine in certain proportions tends to turn Greek wine from red to blue. It was commonplace in Homer's day to mix water and wine.

2. Manfred Lurker, *Gods and Symbols of Ancient Egypt* (Thames & Hudson, 1980).

3. June Osborne, *Stained Glass in England* (Frederick Muller Ltd., London, 1981).

Further reading

Dr R.M.Burke, *Cosmic Consciousness*   (University Books Inc. 1961).

J.C. Cooper, *An Illustrated Encyclopedia of Traditional Symbols* (Thames & Hudson, London, 1978).

Lyall Watson, *Lightning Bird* (Coronet Books, 1982).

Colin Wilson, *Access to Inner Worlds* (Rider, 1983).

2.
Colour In Our Present

Outer Colour and Science

Objectively speaking, there are two main ways by which we are visually aware of colour. We perceive a coloured object by the light reflected from it, and we also see coloured light that comes through transparent matter, such as stained glass, or when a beam of sunlight passes through a prism and white light is split into the colours of the rainbow — red, orange, yellow, green, blue, indigo and violet. Not until 1672 when Sir Isaac Newton described his experiments in passing sunlight through a glass prism was it possible to explain the appearance of the colours of the rainbow. Now we know that visible light is just a very small part of the vast spectrum of radio waves, varying in length and speed, as in the case of visible light — from red, the slowest and longest, to blue, the fastest and shortest.

Before we go into the subject of radio waves however, it might be as well to take a brief look at the mechanism of seeing colour. Without involving too much technical detail, it can be said that the human eye interprets light rays (electro-magnetic energy) by an interaction of the optic nerves with the brain, involving a system of rods and cones in the retina, and externalizes these as colours. It seems that there are about 1000 distinguishable hues and more than 2,000 tints and shades perceived by the human eye. For the colour-blind this is severely limited. Experiments have found that one person out of every fifty-five cannot tell red from green, and one in fifty confuses brown and green. Pink and yellow look alike to some people, and blue and green are similar for others. A very few people see everything in black and white.

Life holds hazards for the colour-blind, who cannot distinguish coloured lights at airports, on ships, and traffic and railway signals, except by guesswork. A friend who was a pilot during the last war said he couldn't understand why Ground Control 'over-reacted' sometimes when he came in to land. It turned out that he couldn't distinguish the red warning light from the green go-ahead. At that time he was in his early 20's and had no idea that he was colour-blind. The red electrical 'live' wire thus holds particular dangers for the colour blind, which is presumably why Common Market regulations have caused it to be changed to brown, with blue for neutral and striped green and yellow for earth.

The various colours are produced by light waves of different lengths. Objects do not possess a fixed colour of their own but depend for colour on the light reflected from their surfaces. Leaves on plants appear green because they reflect green rays and absorb all other light, but if a leaf is held under a red light it will appear black. All things are thus any colour — yellow, blue or brown according to their ability to absorb certain light rays and reflect others. Transparent objects are coloured by their ability to screen out certain rays — as in blue glass, for instance, when only blue rays pass through it. A transparent object which transmits all colours equally well, such as pure water in small quantities, is said to be colourless.

Colours differ in 'hue', which is the difference between blue and red, green and yellow, and colours of the same hue may differ in 'value' or intensity, owing to the difference in the amount of light they reflect; or in 'purity', according to the amount of greyness in the colours. Surfaces capable of reflecting all colour rays appear red in red light, blue in blue light and white in daylight. Other surfaces absorb all light rays and reflect none. These are 'black'. Adding white to a standard hue, as in red becoming pink, 'tints'; while adding black forms 'shades'. Artists' colours and all the other dyes, paints and inks used by man, produce colour because of their ability to reflect different light waves and from just a few substances a great many colours can be created. Blue, red and yellow are called primary colours as from different combinations of these all other colours may be produced.

Colours form complementary pairs such as red and green, yellow and violet, blue and orange. One of the tricks our eyes can play on us is to cause us to see a complementary colour image. This is where, as will be explained in a later chapter, difficulties can arise in 'seeing' the aura. Someone wearing

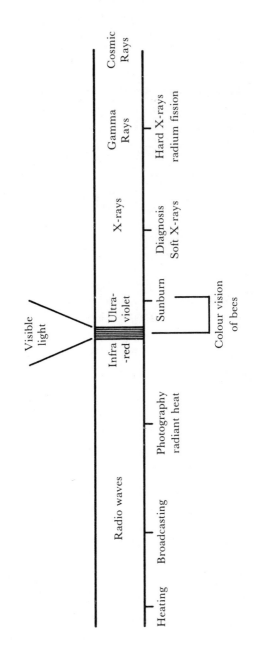

Figure 1: The Electro-Magnetic Spectrum

bright red will often appear to have a green aura around them and so on. If you stare fixedly at a bright green object and then look away quickly at a white surface you will see a replica of the object in red. This is because the eye soon tires of one colour, so that when looking at a white surface or pale background it welcomes the other colours and responds less to the colour that has produced fatigue. In fact, if you stare at anything too fixedly the eye becomes tired and one of the most common colours then seen is a greeny-blue — another point to bear in mind if you are looking at auras.

As mentioned above, visible light is only a very small part of the electro-magnetic spectrum; in fact it covers only 1/60th of the known radio spectrum, as shown in Figure 1.

Long radio waves are used for radio communications, induction heat, photography — where they can penetrate great distance and heavy atmospheres and take pictures where the human eye can hardly see. Next comes radiant heat, laser beams for cutting, and holography. Long waves can measure several thousand feet from crest to crest, whereas the wave length of, say, sodium (yellow) light is very short — about 45,000 waves to an inch. At the far short end of the spectrum are X-rays, gamma rays, and cosmic rays. Most of these rays pass through our bodies harmlessly, although over-exposure to X-rays, gamma rays, microwaves, laser beams, etc. is extremely dangerous, if not lethal. Visible light also penetrates quite a way into animal and human muscle, even as far as the central organs if the light intensity is strong enough. Scientist E.E.Brunt and his associates[1] caused light to penetrate the skulls of sheep, dogs and rabbits and demonstrated 'that light does reach the temporal lobes and hypothalamus in a variety of mammalian species' — no doubt in the human being also. Another scientist, W.F.Ganong and his colleagues concluded that 'environmental light can penetrate the mammalian skull in sufficient amount to activate photoelectric cells embedded in the brain tissue.' 'This means,' says Faber Birren, 'that light is essential to a healthful and normal life and that nature has evolved ways in which it affects the body through the tissues of the skin, the eyes, and even the skull itself.'

The human being and all other creatures also emit light and radiation waves of their own, quite apart from those creatures which have a luminous appearance, such as glow-worms, fireflies and deep-sea fish. Dr Glen Rein, a biologist from St.

Bartholomew's Hospital, London, said in a lecture at the College of Psychic Studies (April 1983) that the human body emits many of the radio waves, including visible light (the latter partly as the aura). Dr Rein has worked with healers and found that healing energy and electromagnetic energy has a significant effect on enzyme activity and neurotransmission. He described how crystals emit an electric current under pressure and how electromagnetic energy can be fed into them. He pointed out that there were crystals in the pineal gland, for instance, and it could be assumed from this that if electromagnetic energy is fed into them in some way it could possibly have profound effects on one's health.

It is therefore evident that not only radio waves but visible light has a significant effect on humans and all other creatures. Even the lower animals such as amoeba react to light, some preferring weak light or shade, or very little light at all. Light has a profound effect on human and animal sexual cycles. For instance, the starlings of Piccadilly who are exposed to all the brilliance of advertisement and street lighting, were found to have active reproductive organs at a time when their country cousins outside the city were sexually impotent. One could of course put it down to the influence of Eros but somehow other scientific tests appear to refute this!

Farmers have found that chickens lay more eggs in winter if extra light is provided, and weasels, rabbits and ferrets have been induced to grow winter fur coloration during the hot days of summer by manipulating the amount of light available to them. In his fascinating book *Light, Color and Environment*, Faber Birren reports that similar results have been achieved with goats, whereby breeding and milk supply can be controlled. Apparently short days induce breeding and long days inhibit it.

Birren also mentions a case study in which mink were reared behind different coloured plastic windows by scientist John Ott.[2] Normally mink are very aggressive, particularly during the mating period. Ott found that mink kept behind pink windows became increasingly aggressive and vicious and there was less frequency of pregnancy after mating. However mink kept behind blue plastic became more docile and could be handled easily. All females became pregnant after mating. It seems also that the human male is excited by red radiation and pacified by blue.

Most mammals are, from our point of view at least, virtually colour-blind although colour vision exists in insects, fish, reptiles, birds and apes. All however react to colour whether they can 'see' it or not. Rodents kept under blue light were found to have normal growth rate but under pink or red appetite increased and subsequently weight. But prolonged exposure to pink resulted in death to mice. John Ott kept 1000 mice in separate colonies with three different forms of lighting — bluish fluorescent, pinkish fluorescent and natural daylight. (Although of course 'natural daylight' can vary greatly in intensity depending on the time of day and season of the year.) He found that under natural light offspring produced were 50 per cent male and 50 per cent female; but under blue light offspring were 70 per cent female and 30 per cent male; and under pink it was 70 per cent male and 30 per cent female! The use of bluish artificial light (presumably in order to breed more females with thicker coats) is commonplace among commercial breeders of chinchilla.

Plants also are significantly affected by light intensity, length of day and colour even more than by temperature and moisture conditions. By the process of photosynthesis, light causes carbon dioxide and water to unite in the presence of chlorophyll to form simple sugars. Most of these are food for the plants as well as for the animals and humans who subsequently eat them.

Birren tells us that Tessier of France[3] (1783) was one of the pioneers investigating growth of plants by means of coloured light and he recorded marked growth differences. Then later General A.J.Pleasanton of Philadelphia upset the horticultural applecart by propounding various startling theories regarding the use of blue (which he regarded as the most important colour) glass panes in his greenhouse. He claimed great yields of grapes with this system although Birren feels these were exaggerated. In 1895, C.Flammarion reported best effects with red light, and in 1902 L.C.Corbett found that red light had a markedly stimulating effect on lettuce growth. These and various other investigators have been followed by more scientifically orientated experimenters.

It is standard practice now amongst many gardeners to regulate the amount of light their plants receive. John Ott found that chrysanthemums could be made to flower any month of the year by regulating their exposure to light. He carried out many experiments also with coloured light and filters. He found that the male and female flowers of the pumpkin, for instance, reacted to bluish daylight fluorescent light by respectively withering and flourishing. Regular fluorescent light caused the female flowers to wither but not the male. Blue light and filters caused morning glory to open but warm light shrivelled them up. It would seem therefore that by taking careful note of the time of year and prevailing conditions in which a plant flourishes, it should in theory be possible to grow almost anything out of its normal season and environment, except that to my mind something grown 'out of season' never has the flavour or texture of naturally grown vegetables and fruit. Even so the effects of light and colour on plants are most intriguing and a wonderful example of the interaction of various forces combining to produce the world we live in.

It appears that like other organisms, plants are most responsive to red and blue, and inactive to yellow and yellow-green. Red will cause lettuce seed to sprout, but infra-red will send the sprouts to sleep again. Red will also inhibit flowering of short day plants (presumably autumn or winter plants) and assist flowering of long day (late spring and summer) plants. If one works for any length of time in an illuminated greenhouse then weak green illumination is best for both human eyes and also for the plants, as it does not cause any adverse reaction from either. Stuart Dunn of the University of New Hampshire found that tomato seeds produced interesting results when grown under different coloured lamps. Warm white lamps produced the highest yield (this is probably comparable to natural sunlight). Next came blue and pink lamps. Green and red were low while experimental 'high intensity' red lamps produced the highest yield of all. Nowadays special lamps are available to growers wishing to get their plants off to an early start.

Theo Gimbel[4] found that primary red filter light initially overstimulated plant growth, which later became stunted, with an elastic texture and bitter taste. Green started off well but ultimately disintegrated. Those under a blue filter did even better than those under clear light, growing thickly and higher than had been anticipated. He does not however name the plants grown, so it might be as well to be a little cautious if you are thinking of trying out blue filters on any exotic seeds which you may have acquired, as they might well require a different type of light altogether.

Another interesting point is revealed by Birren, who points

out that 'some plant life has an aura!' Apparently in 1923 Alexander Gurwitsch[5] wrote of discovering what he called 'mitogenetic energy', whereby an onion, for example, emits rays in the shorter ultra-violet region of the spectrum. Although of very low intensity it has tangible and measurable existence. This has been verified by subsequent investigators but is still something of a mystery with various scientists holding completely opposing opinions.

Faber Birren, who might be described as the Grand Old Man of colour research and who has hundreds of articles and many books published on colour and its implications, cites many interesting pieces of research on the effects of light and colour on the human organism. He quotes H.L.Logan, a leading lighting engineer who points out that light dilates blood vessels, increases circulation, and thus rids of the body of toxins and lightens the load on the kidneys. Haemoglobin in the blood will be increased by light and decreased by darkness. Light also induces hormonal processes through the activation of endocrine glands. Another researcher, Richard J. Wurtman, has evidence that the stimulation of light may come through the eyes, but can also trigger effects through the skin and subcutaneous tissues. He states: 'it seems clear that light is the most important environmental input, after food, in controlling bodily function.'

Wurtman also found that blind girls tended to menstruate earlier than girls with normal vision and thought it possible that this was due to the fact that 'in the absence of retinal response to light (this) produces an imbalance which results in earlier menstrual function.' Among Eskimo women menstruation may cease during the long arctic night and here possibly lack of light leads to a natural form of human hibernation.

We can thus understand that colour and light affect the whole of life. How effective then are the claims for healing by colour? In this chapter we shall examine some of the more orthodox claims for colour therapy since the days of Niels R. Finsen. Niels R. Finsen of Denmark was the pioneer of light research. He believed that visible red light would prevent scar formation in cases of smallpox and in 1896 he wrote of the actinic (chemical action) properties of sunlight and founded a Light Institute for the cure of tuberculosis. He was awarded a Nobel Prize in 1903 and later reported startling cures among some 2000 patients, using both sunlight and ultraviolet light. Birren tells us that Downs and Blunt of England discovered in 1877 the bactericidal action of ultraviolet radiation. In India rickets is fairly common, which may be due to the custom of women and children in higher castes staying indoors most of the day, but there is also an incidence of rickets when people of sunnier climates come to Britain and are similarly deprived of sunshine and vitamin D. Ultraviolet radiation is essential — it produces vitamin D, prevents rickets, destroys germs, and effects certain necessary chemical changes in the body and can be used to cure various skin diseases.

In the United States ultraviolet has become standard treatment for psoriasis. Fish in aquariums can be cured of some virus diseases by radiating them with a certain amount of ultraviolet light. It works equally well for other animals. It can also be used for irradiating foodstuffs such as lard, oil, and milk to form vitamin D but oddly enough cod-liver oil loses its main properties after irradiation. Ulraviolet radiation also tends to increase protein metabolism and helps reduce sugar level in the blood of diabetics. However short term over-exposure can cause skin damage and a painful eye condition known as photokeratitis. Long term effects include skin cancers and cataracts of the eyes. Infra-red long waves are very hazardous to the human eye and also seem to have a deleterious effect on the action of vitamin D.

There are many scientists who are convinced that colour, as well as light, has a more powerful impact on health and behaviour than previously thought and colour is used nowadays in treating a variety of diseases. For instance, within the last 10-15 years, baths of blue light have replaced blood transfusions for about 30,000 premature babies born each year with potentially fatal neonatal jaundice (U S figures). However, blue lights irritate the nurses working in these wards and many hospitals have added gold lamps to impart a soothing quality.[6] In general it has been found that working with babies is greatly helped by blue light, which lessens crying and over-activity.

White fluorescent light, in conjunction with photosensitizing drugs, is widely used to help heal herpes sores. Some unlucky people develop a skin rash if exposed to visible blue or violet light — this may be due to aftershave lotions, cosmetics etc. or the allergic effect of eating certain foods or by handling allergy-creating substances which interact with light. Nowadays there are effective drugs to counteract unwanted radiation. Certain dyes are also used on such conditions as psoriasis and herpes which are then exposed to visible light. In this way visible light can help heal damage caused by invisible ultraviolet light. One dye, chrome yellow, has been found particularly effective[7] when used in conjunction with a blue-violet light source. The use of porphyrins (sensitizing agents) has had favourable effects on some minor forms of cancer and tumours, whereby they accumulate at the afflicted area and any cancerous tissue, for example, is 'severely damaged when exposed to visible or near ultraviolet light'. The use of dyes and light for skin afflictions is still at a very controversial stage and many scientists do not consider them useful.

In Soviet Russia, where for some considerable time they have been experimenting with and using colour therapy, extensive use is made of ultraviolet, particularly in cases where they suspect miners might be susceptible to black lung disease. They also use it to supplement schoolroom light. As a result it is claimed that children grow faster than usual, with fewer colds and improved work performances.

Some investigators working on the effects of colour on bodily activities claim that red light increases muscular activity, blood pressure, respiration and heart rate. In fact red appears to be a very disturbing colour for anxious persons. Blue has the reverse effect, reducing blood-pressure and eyeblink frequency and subsequently any eye irritations, and is thought to be conducive to sleep. Red might be useful in arousing persons troubled with reactive depression or neurasthenia. In some instances it seems to improve growth. It also causes a decrease in blood sugar and has been recommended for some cases of eczema. Gestalt psychologists such as Heinz Werner, Krakov, Allen and Schwartz have found that loud noises, strong odours and tastes, tend to raise the sensitivity of the eye to green, and to decrease sensitivity to red. Birren states 'It may thus be generalized that colour affects muscular tension, cortical activation (brain waves), heart rate, respiration, and other functions of the autonomic nervous system.'

It may affect someone even more dramatically — Birren tells of a woman with a cerebellar disease who had a tendency to fall unexpectedly. When she wore a red dress such symptoms were more pronounced. He points out that tremor and some conditions of Parkinson's Disease 'can at times be diminished in severity if the individuals are protected against red or yellow, if they wear, for instance, spectacles with green lenses. Those wishing to pursue these ideas in greater depth are recommended to study the books of Faber Birren.

While most colour studies have been from the psychological point of view some doctors are beginning to realise that the eye needs moderate contrast and variety if it is to function well. Hospitals, which are rather emotive places, are choosing soothing colours for waiting rooms and wards. When one recalls the early days of grim antiseptic surroundings in hospitals and similar institutions one is thankful that most of them nowadays at least make an effort towards a cheerier environment. As said before, brightness and vividness of colour tend to arouse autonomic functions, blood-pressure, heart and respiration rate. Dimness and softness of colour tend to have reverse effects and to invite repose. Autonomic functions are retarded and there is more inner relaxation.

In surgery, the problem of glare from high intensity lights has led to the use of turquoise and blue-green in surroundings as well as for garments; this reduces brightness in the field of view, builds up better visual contrast and obviates the problem of the surgeon being distracted by green after-images from blood. For patients, soft tones, not too highly reflective, are best. Ceilings should perhaps be tinted in view of the fact that some patients have to lie and gaze at them. Brilliant colours such as reds, yellows and blues may not only prove monotonous for long-term patients but in the case of a disease such as jaundice, a yellow room would make a patient look ten times worse! For such cases uniform lighting is important so that any change in a patient can be quickly noticed. Brighter colours in day and recreation rooms may however be advantageous.

In overall studies of colour preferences and association of colour, the three most appealing are blue, red and green (in all their tints and variations) and the three least appealing are orange, purple, and yellow-green. Blue is better in tones of aquamarine and turquoise as large areas of it tend to have a cold and bleak look. In short, cool, subdued colours are more suitable for chronic patients, while warm, bright colours are better for convalescent patients. Birren recommends that treatment rooms could be coral, peach, light green or aqua, and coral for a nursery. Visitors rooms should be soft yellow, or with a contrasting wall for eye interest.

Hazel Rossotti in her book *Colour*[8] relates how disturbed children in a residential home were asked to paint a picture. A note was taken of the dominant colour in each picture and this colour was subsequently painted on the screen around each individual cubicle. When the children went to bed this seemed to settle them down for the night in a relaxed fashion. Patients at a mental hospital were found more likely to venture along a corridor painted dark purple, brown or crimson than if it were painted a lighter colour; the oppressive effect of the darker colours forced them to look for a more peaceful abode.

One of the most dramatic and controversial developments is the use of the 'pink room' for calming violent people.[9] At the San Bernardino County Probation Department in California, aggressive and violent children are put in an 8ft. × 4ft. cell with one distinctive feature — it is bubble gum pink. According to the director of clinical services, Paul E. Boccumini, after ten minutes or so the children calm down, stop yelling and banging, and tend to fall asleep. What is more important, the effect lasts for some time. There are psychologists who are very sceptical of this treatment but many local authorities in the U S are experimenting with passive pink in the hope of eliminating vandalism and graffiti, while football coaches try the colour in visitors' dressing rooms in the hope that their opponents will come over all lethargic! Whatever psychologists say, we all know that an entirely pink room does have a rather weird effect, inducing drowsiness and inertia.

Theo Gimbel, in his book *Healing Through Colour*,[10] mentions the calming down of a violent crowd by Gerrard and Hessey in 1932 by using blue light, and suggests that cricket matches may be more peaceful than football because they are played in the open air rather than under arc lights. He also tells of a London exhibition in 1970 where three rooms were individually painted in black, green and yellow. For some reason the only room where objects were continually stolen or broken was the yellow room and from this it was concluded that people didn't like yellow. Yellow, in Gimbel's opinion, is a colour which provokes violence and generates a feeling of detachment and non-involvement. He suggests the possibility that yellow street lights may have some relevance to the incidence of crime in an area.

Schools also are trying to get away from the strictly functional image of earlier years and tend to go in for sometimes quite exotic colour schemes and brilliant murals (although whether this is appreciated by the pupils is another matter). What is important is the way that the modern principles of colour applied to schools will improve the scholastic performance of students, especially so in their earlier years. There is always the possibility, of course, that schoolchildren` who are at the receiving end of 'experiments' in colour may react positively simply due to the fact that interesting things are happening around them and attention is being paid to them, as has been found the case with factory workers in a dull environment, whose production will shoot up when 'experts' are called in to brighten up the surroundings. However from the purely physical point of view a background should be chosen which does not harm the eyes or distract attention — glare from too-white walls and poor visibility are both to be avoided. Light colours reflect more illumination than dark ones but too much brightness is a handicap, creating a visible 'pull' away from books and tasks. Ceilings, Birren advises, should be white for good light reflection and for floors natural wood is ideal. Bright, warm colours are best for younger children and places of relaxation — soft yellow, coral, peach, etc. The more passive effect of chartreuse, (a pale yellowy-green), light green or aqua will allow better concentration. Hence cool colours become appropriate for upper grades and study rooms and libraries. End wall colour treatments are particularly appropriate to schools, where a neutral shade would be suitable for the three walls not facing the students, and a more colourful contrasting shade such as terracotta, old gold, avocado, turquoise or blue would break up the monotony by giving the classroom a different appearance from different directions. Gymnasiums, manual training and domestic science rooms are probably best in luminous tones of soft yellow, peach, beige, while canteens and dining rooms should be in cheerful and 'appetizing' colours such as peach, coral, rose, pumpkin and flamingo. All obstacles should be painted bright yellow or red so that they draw the eye.

Inner Colour and Nature
Another way in which we can experience colour is subjectively, from inside ourselves. Ever since Huxley's experiments with mescaline, many people have tried out such drugs as LSD, Peyote and even more dangerous substances. Some of these experiments have been conducted along scientific lines, purely for research; others purely for self-indulgence or through misguided curiosity, without the safeguards used by doctors or by those who have used them traditionally as a means of

spiritual seeking. What probably set off most people were the descriptions given by Huxley and others of the extraordinary visual effects, especially those involving colour. Huxley himself was particularly impressed by the enhanced sense of colour awareness after taking mescaline and many more since then have given even more titillating descriptions of the effects produced by these drugs. Strobe lamps are said to enhance one's visualization of colour and while from personal experience, I can say that for some hours after being subjected to a brief encounter with a strobe lamp, my subjective visualization of colour certainly seemed much easier to achieve, I do not really see the point of it! Strobe lamps can be dangerous if not properly regulated and in the hands of the inexperienced can cause epileptic attacks or migraine. A less dangerous way of subjective colour experience involves the use of the 'Black Box' where a person is cut off from all forms of sensory perception. After some hours spent entombed in one of these rooms, most people experience some form of hallucination, often involving dazzling colour displays. In fact often before an attack of epilepsy or migraine the sufferer will see coloured rays or zig-zag patterns before, or at the side of, his eyes. Again if one gets a thump on the head or in the eye, a remarkable display of shooting stars will be experienced! Colours are also experienced vividly in dreams and meditations and this will be discussed in a later chapter.

In his book, *Access to Inner Worlds*,[11] Colin Wilson mentions a very unusual work *Essay on the Origin of Thought* by Jurij Moskvitin. In it the author describes how one day, lying in the sunlight with eyes half-closed, he was observing the colour spectrum that sometimes becomes visible when the eyelashes partly screen the eyes. He then says, 'Suddenly I became aware as if of a film in the background, a screen or mosaic with the most strange and beautiful patterns which gave me the feeling of watching something particularly significant.' He later became convinced that these patterns were made of 'dancing sparks' and compared the effect to a painting by pointillist painter Signac. He began to believe that our normal vision is made up of these sparks. Colin Wilson's interpretation of Moskvitin's rather obscure ideas is that he is saying that 'the external world our eyes reveal to us is just a limited version of that larger inner world.' In other words, 'Seeing is an instantaneous act of painting, and the paintbrush is this magical rush of 'sparks' from our eyes.'

Yet another way of subjectively 'seeing' colour is by using other parts of the body than our eyes. It has been found that many blind people develop a colour sense by running their fingertips over a surface and gaining the impression that one colour is warm, another cool and acid, another heavy and thick, and so on. It's quite fun to try this for yourself with colour cards.

Most research on this seems to have been undertaken in the Soviet Union and in *Psychic Discoveries Behind the Iron Curtain*[12] by Ostrander and Schroeder, a chapter is devoted to 'Eyeless Sight.' The most famous exponent of this ability is Rosa Kuleshova, who was not only able to 'see' colours when blindfolded, but also to read print and distinguish pictures simply by touching them with her hands. She said it took several hours a day of practice and almost overnight she became a celebrity. Russians took to 'the great eyeless sight fad' with immense enthusiasm and unfortunately the same sort of hysteria gripped the nation as 'metal-bending' did in Britain in the wake of Yuri Geller, and somewhat discredited the subject. But in the background scientists tried to uncover the mechanics of this unusual ability. It was first thought that Rosa was supersensitive to the texture of dye but she was able, after being securely blindfolded and behind a thick cardboard screen, to identify red, green and yellow even when tracing paper, cellophane or glass covered the colour sheets. So they then thought she might be supersensitive to heat and so used heated plates with cool colours and *vice versa*. But this didn't make any difference. She was also able to identify coloured liquids in a glass tube. Using both hands Rosa was able to 'see' the colour of anything from a tie to a postage stamp. From consulting old records it was found that other people also had this ability. One doctor at the Nizhniy Tagil Pedagogical Institute found that about every sixth person could tell the difference between two colours after about half an hour's practice. Most people agreed that colours divide into smooth, sticky, and rough sensations — light blue being smoothest, yellow as very slippery. Red, green and dark blue are 'sticky', while violet was very sticky and rough. Not everyone 'sees' colour like this — Rosa herself sensed various colours as crosses, straight lines, dots, etc.

Dr Novomeisky, who undertook most of these experiments, believes eyeless sight has something to do with electromagnetic fields. He tried putting the colour cards in an insulated tray and his students began to react as if the colour extended some way above the tray into space. Different people sensed colours at differing heights but all took similar steps up the colour spectrum — red extended highest for everyone and blue extended least. Then further experiments were carried out with sightless people by beaming coloured light onto their palms and eventually this was extended to the outlines of letters. Today eyeless sight is called 'bio-introscopy' and as further experiments are being carried out, perhaps it may develop into an ability which can be aquired by most sightless people.

The Soviets say that all one's skin has seeing potential and report trainees sensing light and colour with the tongue, elbow and nose. One wonders if this also could be extended to the senses of taste, hearing and smell. Many claims have also come out of China regarding children able to 'see' with their elbows, stomachs, knees, etc. It is a fascinating subject but how much is due to the 'experimenter effect' is open to debate. The 'experimenter effect' is an increasingly common explanation of a phenomenon whereby the experimenter is thought to be unconsciously influencing his subjects, as often the experiments in question are not able to be repeated by others.

Let us now turn from the somewhat sterile world of science to the natural everyday life around us. Many brilliant colour effects in nature are not chemical in origin. The rainbow and similar manifestations — the iridescence of oil on water, soap bubbles, birds' feathers, etc. — are phenomena of light caused by refraction, polarization and so on. Many non-metallic colours found in birds' wings, for example, are formed by small air bubbles in the feathers that cause white rays to split apart into their component colours. A similar process occurs through interference of light rays as they pass through the thin layers of wing in butterflies, dragonflies and various beetles. Nothing is quite what it seems. Even the lustre of mother-of-pearl is caused by light defraction. Such manifestations as sunrise and sunset are caused by scattered light and if there are heavy dust particles in the atmosphere, this can account for some spectacular effects. Light scattering also accounts for blue eyes, blue feathers, and the highly decorative rear end of the mandrill baboon. In fact light scattering accounts for a lot of colouring in nature and this, as said before, can be caused by tiny air spaces. Most colours come about by absorption or selective reflection, whereby say a 'red' surface absorbs most of the rays at the blue end of the spectrum and reflects back the remainder — the red!

It is therefore an interesting thought that when we are looking at a person of another colour, we are really only looking at someone whose skin has the ability to absorb certain colour rays and reject others. Even so, certain ailments can cause the skin to change colour dramatically. Perspiration can change colour under stress, as in 1709 when an unfortunate girl turned 'dark as a negress' when under stress, and was accused of witchcraft. In the animal world, hippopotami, for example, exude red perspiration.

Many insects, animals, fish and reptiles change their colours according to the environment, time of year, even the time of day. Crabs and shrimps for instance adapt their colouring to their environment, their skin being covered in pigment cells which are stimulated through the eyes to effect the necessary colour change. Tropical fish in particular undergo very interesting colour changes, often for no obvious reason. And of course the chameleon is well-known for its colour-changing abilities, being extremely sensitive to light. This appears to be regulated through its eyes. Many other creatures use their colour as defence camouflage, or to disguise themselves in wait for prey; others flaunt brilliant 'poisonous' colours to deceive an intending predator.

Nature displays a vast ingenuity in arranging colour effects — like placing small lens-like structures in mosses to make them gleam; producing iridescence and fluoresence in seaweed, moulds and fungi; luminesence in the ocean (often caused by bacteria) or in such living creatures as corals. Birren tells us that much has been discovered about the luminous organs of deep-sea creatures. 'Some have organs like eyes, which emit light.' Nearly all are luminous or have luminous spots, often coloured — in fact some sound like outer-space craft, with rows of green, red and orange spots. Certain others become luminous at mating time, but otherwise luminosity may be for attracting prey or frightening hostile predators, or even so that like may recognise like.

Going from the sea to the sky, the colour and variety of stars seems infinite, planets and suns being quite easily identifiable as blue, red, gold, etc. Sirius, for example, is one of the most colourful stars seen in the winter skies in the northern hemisphere, flashing and sparkling in rainbow colours. Also there is the aurora, that spectacular display of dancing lights at the poles, prosaically caused by the bombardment of air by electrons and other particles which stream in from the sun in great quantity and at great speed.

Much on our earth is affected colourwise by the time of day, season of the year and weather conditions, when the quality of light changes dramatically from dawn to dusk. This in turn subtly affects all life, regulates procreation and growth, slows down and speeds up all processes in the human and non-human kingdoms. Even the colour of soil varies tremendously according to the various minerals present in it. Stone, rock and sand, even ordinary-looking pebbles, have a beauty of their own when examined closely. Hazel Rossotti[13] tells us that some of the most beautiful colours of the mineral world are caused by optical interference. For instance, opal absorbs little visible light, being made up almost entirely of silica and water and in fact acts as a diffraction grating. Depending on the angle of viewing, light of one or more wavelengths is cancelled out, and thus the opal appears to change its colours continuously. Cut diamonds spread light far more effectively than say a dewdrop or a glass prism, the various colours emerging at different angles according to how the diamond is faceted. Other gems owe their colour to various minerals and ores present in their structure, which in turn absorb some rays and reflect others. Again, as the makers of fireworks well know, chemical elements have their characteristic fire colours — a green flame for copper and pale mauve for potassium, for example, and this is evident in the variety and colour of fire in all its aspects.

Thus the four elements of earth, air, fire and water give us endless examples of the effect of colour and the interaction of light with everything from oxygen particles to minute water bubbles. Earth has its flowers, fruits, rocks and human and animal life in great colourful profusion; air provides us with splendid sun and sky effects; while water, ever-changing, offers an endless interplay of light and subtle colour.

References

1.   Faber Birren, *Light, Color and the Environment* (Van Nostrand Reinhold Co.Inc., 1969).

2. Faber Birren, *Color and Human Response* (Van Nostrand Reinhold Co.Inc., 1978).
3. Faber Birren, *Color: a Survey in Words and Pictures* (University Books, N.Y., 1963).
4. Theo Gimbel, *Healing Through Colour* (The C.W.Daniel Co.Ltd., 1980).
5. Faber Birren, *Color and Human Response* (Van Nostrand Reinhold Co.Inc., 1978).
6. 'Science Times' *New York Times*, October 19, 1982.
7. Faber Birren, *Color and Human Response* (Van Nostrand Reinhold Co.Inc., 1978).
8. Hazel Rossotti, *Colour: Why the World Isn't Grey* (Pelican Books, 1983).
9. 'Science Times' *New York Times*, October 19, 1982.
10. Theo Gimbel, *Healing Through Colour* (The C.W.Daniel Co.Ltd., 1980).
11. Colin Wilson, *Access to Inner Worlds* (Rider, 1983).
12. Sheila Ostrander & Lynn Schroeder, *Psychic Discoveries Behind the Iron Curtain*, (Sphere Books, 1973).
13. Hazel Rossotti, *Colour: Why the World Isn't Grey* (Pelican Books, 1983).

3
Colour In Our Living

1. Exterior Colour

Place of work

Most people may not think they notice the colours that assail them from all sides in their everyday environment — one's general surroundings, other people's dress, brightly coloured advertisements — it all seems to pass by as a blur. But we still react fairly sharply and our eyes and body have registered a particular colour often long before our conscious self is aware of it.

In that environment where perforce we spend most of our days, our place of work, unless we are particularly fortunate we tend to be surrounded by drab shades of beige, cream and dirty grey. Luckily most large organizations are becoming a little more colour conscious, realizing that a depressing background makes for depressed workers. Clearly though, as *action* is usually required at places of work it wouldn't do to have a soporific background and too many soft, warm lights about the place.

Much depends on the type of work to be undertaken. Colour improperly applied can interfere with tasks, distract from work and cause much eye-strain. If one is an office worker, for example, a neutral and non-distracting cool colour helps to keep the eye at a comfortable level of adjustment. The desk should also be in a neutral shade — grey for instance reduces the effect of blinking and thus reduces fatigue. When workers glance up their eyes should rest on a pleasing, relaxing colour such as blue, green or turquoise. Too much white causes glare and constricts pupil opening but deep colours can open the eyes too wide and lead to eye fatigue. Soft clear colours, with possibly a contrast wall, are best. White is very tiresome to look at if one suffers from 'sleepers' in the eye — a white page such as this provides ample opportunity for them to appear. Also, in glancing from a strong colour to white, one always gets a distracting after-image. Deep or strong colours should never be put on window walls but are best placed on walls behind desks, or on walls facing people. Good colours for offices, study rooms, fine assembly in industry are the cool hues — grey, blue, green, turquoise. There is thus less outer distraction and a person can concentrate on precision work.

On the other hand if you work in a factory or workshop where there is much manual activity, brighter colours around the place may be more helpful. Over the last few decades most industrial plants have made a great effort to improve lighting and introduce various colour schemes in the hope of inspiring their workers to greater effort. As with office workers, those workers who have to undertake intricate tasks need to rest their eyes on a pleasing, non-distracting colour when they look up. Whilst it is not possible within the scope of this book to enter into any great detail as regards colour schemes for business and industrial units, a few major priorities should be mentioned. Faber Birren suggests in several of his books a colour scheme he has devised for factories and much of this now seems standard practice in the more advanced industrial complexes. Most are common sense — machinery should be highlighted with pale colours to reflect more light on the important parts; vivid yellow and black bands should be used to emphasize hazards and obstructions; vivid orange for acute hazards likely to cause harm or shock; brilliant green for all first aid equipment; vivid red for firefighting equipment; vivid blue as a standard caution signal. White, grey and black are suggested for traffic control. Last but not least he recommends that corners should be painted white to discourage litter and to catch the eye of the sweeper. Many of these ideas have been adopted in rail, road and other public service systems.

Another area in factories and offices which has been long neglected is the washroom, usually painted in dire shades no doubt in the hope that one will not be tempted to linger. But as men seem to prefer blue and women pink or coral, it would be appreciated by workers if these dreary places could be brightened up a little with at least a touch of these colours. Cafeterias and canteens can also be fairly dismal, and here appetizing colours — the 'warm' colours, or pleasantly fresh, cool hues, can help in achieving a relaxed meal break.

Shopping and eating out

Nowadays there is every sort of shop for every sort of customer and a subsequent thriving industry in colour and décor arrangement devoted to bringing customers in. Even so, we have probably all had the experience of entering a café or shop and immediately recoiling because of the unfavourable impression it gives. Perhaps some people don't mind buying clothes in a shop where the colour scheme and lighting makes them look like something out of the Chamber of Horrors, or eating their meal in Dante's Inferno! I remember a meal in what seemed like a delightful little restaurant where the lighting was so poor that everything we ate looked dark brown. I wouldn't go there again.

The same applies to clothes and food shops. Poor lighting and indifferent colour schemes do not encourage people to buy and owners of such places may wonder why they are not doing good business. Sensible shopkeepers try to align their colour scheme to their wares. Most men's shops are decorated in dignified, dark warm colours which give the impression of a discreet 'Men's club' atmosphere. The shopkeepers know full well that most of their customers are fairly conservative and wouldn't appreciate anything 'feminine' or trendy. However a different colour scheme applies to women's shops, for conditioned as we are from birth to accept certain colours as feminine and others as masculine, most of us like to buy our clothes in 'pretty' or 'opulent' surroundings.

Unfortunately most clothes shops and large stores don't seem to understand that a cold, white light won't help their sales. Anywhere that customers have to see themselves in a mirror would do better to go for warm, low intensity lighting, as this will be in most of their homes. According to Birren, the most flattering background colour for complexions is turquoise and this is ideal for clothes shops and beauty parlours. A white background tends to dull the complexion; red drains it of pinkness and lime green turns it purple! While sitting under a hairdryer in the hairdressers does tend to turn one's face puce, it's surprising the number of hairdressers who still use poor lighting and unflattering background colours, which doesn't help.

When shopping for food we tend to have idealistic colour memories and many foods are tinted because we always remember them as more colourful than they really are. Given two jars of peas, most people will choose the tinted one. Butter is coloured to give it that rich, golden 'dairy-fresh' look; jams have to appear as if the fruit has just been picked. Some colours are 'sweet' and others 'savoury' and if foods are coloured out of context it generally diminishes our appetite immediately. Wines are liked in golden yellow, deep red and pink — this reminds us of lush bunches of grapes hanging on the vine. Pink or blue bread would not be very popular because we have that vision of golden brown loaves made from ripened wheat. Colours such as mauve and yellow-green can cause nausea and sickness and are not very good choices for food shops or restaurants. Here again turquoise is a good colour for the display of food — meat looks redder and other foods stand out well.

Advertisers play on all these associations, suggesting to us that various foods are 'harvest fresh' and bursting with natural vitamins, while in reality they are probably heavily tinted to induce just that reaction. Bright and warm colours are the appetizers and these are good in restaurants, especially those that wish to encourage people to linger; others wanting a quicker turnover of customers should go for something cooler like blue or green. The colour of plates and tablecloths also plays a great part in presenting food attractively and most pastel shades are suitable.

Home

From shopping and eating out we return to our own homes and this is where we can express our own personalities. A few guidelines can be given for home decoration but it is infinitely preferable for one to make one's own choice. It is no good having a colour scheme just because it is fashionable — *you* have to live with it. There are various booklets in furnishing shops which offer suggestions for particular types of room — although it is important that you give a room the stamp of your own personality. Many of the specially devised layouts in these professionally arranged rooms seem very bland to me, or else claustrophobic, with curtains and wallpaper in the same profuse pattern.

Firstly, you have to take into account such factors as the use of the room, whether it faces in a warm or cool direction, how much sun it gets, and whether you want a peaceful, relaxing room or something a little more stimulating. If you want a soothing colour scheme for say a bedroom, then pale colours, soft warm pinks or apricot, or cooler blues and greens, or mixtures of these, would be appropriate. If you want colourful curtains and cushions then a neutral background is best but remember that white can be tiring for the eyes. For activity rooms like the kitchen, more stimulating colours may appeal — unless of course you tend to be temperamental whilst cooking, in which case cooler hues may be very necessary!

Dark, narrow rooms need light, sunshiny colours; and while coloured ceilings can be oppressive in small rooms, in a large or high room they are very helpful in bringing a ceiling 'down'. But don't overdo any one colour. I once saw a drawing room decorated entirely in blue, with the final touch of a beautiful blue shawl flung over a grand piano; the effect was magnificent but decidedly chilly. Conversely, a room with lots of red may irritate some people, or too much green depress them. Strive for a balance of say one key colour with some of its complementaries in various tints and shades. Don't overdo strong colours, nor let yourself fall into the trap of getting together a mass of colours 'that go with anything' — you'll end up with a sludgy beige room!

If you are outgoing, then your home will probably display bright, warm colours, perhaps with modern furniture and jazzy patterns. If you are quieter, you will probably go for a more traditional effect, with cool, restrained colours. But don't try to change your nature by taking advice from others to 'be bold' or 'more subtle,' otherwise you may feel most unhappy with colours that are not 'you'. Excitable people are not necessarily better off with subdued colours, as they can make them feel bottled up; likewise quieter folk can feel very irritated in brash, trendy surroundings. Small children, who generally like bright colours, are often more tense and difficult in a too-peaceful environment. Here cheerful colours relieve nervousness by creating an outward stimulus to balance the inner high spirits. But often to put a sad, depressed person in too-bright surroundings only makes them retreat even further into their shell.

We must decide for ourselves whether we prefer a bright and colourful environment, or a cool and peaceful one — why not have both in your home? Just remember that warm and luminous colours — yellow, peach, pink — tend to direct the attention outwards, increase general alertness and physical activity. They are good colours for anywhere manual tasks are performed. We are to some extent conditioned by our culture and upbringing in our colour choices — for instance, Latin peoples like bright, warm colours and Nordic peoples the cool, restrained colours. In the temperate zone we fall between the two and thus have plenty of scope. Some people are keen on the great outdoors and like to recreate a forest glade in their homes, with green carpets and blue ceilings, while others go for a more cosy effect, a warm 'cave,' conveying an impression of comfort and security. Others like strictly utilitarian bathrooms and kitchens in functional primary colours, or even black and white. Persons of a more sybaritic disposition may prefer sea-grotto bathrooms, and country kitchens out of old Provence, redolent of herbs and baking bread.

Whatever your choice, remember that colours seem more intense in large areas than small and that colour cards are often very deceptive. If in doubt when covering a large area, aim for a lighter shade than the colour card shows. For example, a pale luminous shade like yellow will be most deceptive on a card but if you dilute the paint with up to 50 per cent white then the colour of the card and the wall will look very much the same. If you like brilliant colours have them on one wall only (not the window end) and you won't be depriving yourself! If you prefer deep colours note that in an artificially lit room they will probably be fine during the day, but at night they have a way of crowding in on one, causing feelings of oppression.

Clothes

The same can be said for clothes as for decorating your home — it's a matter of personal preference and common sense. There are the usual fashion tips about the pale colours making large people look larger, and dark colours narrowing thin people down even more; and that bright colours 'push out' and subtler shades recede. But if a large, extrovert person likes wearing bright colours, why shouldn't they? They won't feel happy if they force themselves into something dull and receding. We all have to wear dull clothes at times, for reasons of expediency, our work and so on, but it shouldn't become a permanent state. If you can't afford to refurbish your wardrobe, then a bright scarf or tie will give the outside world the impression that at least you're alive and kicking! With today's fashions of course almost anything goes, though there are still some rather unlovely results of people adopting fashion too slavishly, but here again it may be that this is the effect they want to achieve. There is plenty of scope to experiment with unusual colours, so don't be limited to 'the colour of your eyes' and try something totally different for a change.

It is a surprising fact that while nowadays clothes are available quite cheaply, often even those who can afford better things pay little attention to colour harmony in their dress, either wearing the same drab mixtures or mixing colours with no regard for a balanced effect. It makes the world a brighter place if everyone dresses a little more adventurously — and it may well affect the wearer also! I am not suggesting that we all go around as if arrayed for a wedding, but we can give a little thought as to the effect of one colour against another, how they detract or add something to each other and whether the general effect is pleasing. Too many people seem to feel that drab, dreary clothes are a mark of modest and self-effacing natures; or else adopt an unhealthy 'I'm drab anyway, so I'll wear drab clothes'. This reveals an exhausted state of mind, rejecting colour as being all too much in a complex world. A little effort here to introduce some upliftment may well help the wearer immensely, for instead of being faced in the mirror with their usual lack-lustre reflection, their eyes will be drawn to that cheerful scarf or tie, and this will have a pleasing and cheering effect.

There are those of course who deliberately cultivate the 'Earth-Mother' or 'Son of the Soil' look, forgetting that Mother Earth goes in for some fairly brilliant colour effects. Punk fashions may not be to everyone's taste but no-one can accuse them of being dreary. While the outside world generally judges us by our appearance, sensible folk know that this is not always an accurate assessment. Even so, the way we dress does portray something of our inward nature and our attitude to the world at large. If we dress carelessly and untidily it not only suggests something of contempt for ourselves but also for our fellow beings, unless of course we belong in the ranks of those elevated thinkers who consider that undue interest in dress is a sign of superficiality of mind and an excessive concern with worldly matters.

Basically, if you like quiet clothes, then be quietly elegant but wear that odd warm colour sometimes. If you like very bright colours, try something subtle for a change. It might make other people look again — even if it's a mistake, at least you've registered!

2. Interior Colour

Colour associations
If we dislike a certain colour it may be that we associate it with some unpleasant or frightening memory, something perhaps long forgotten. Old superstitions die hard; green is still considered unlucky by many people and someone 'looking green' is nauseated. Again, 'green' also means immaturity and naïvety. But it is usually the connotations with the 'Faery Folk' and it being *their* colour that gives green its reputation of ill-luck.

We may like a colour in one texture or form and not in another. You might like purple velvet but detest purple cars. Which brings us to 'purple prose', and the saying 'born in the purple'; also, 'purple with rage', all of which have somewhat different meanings.

As said before, we associate colours with warmth and coolness and people tend to fall in one or another of these groups. But this can be a case of our eyes deceiving us because there is no difference between say a red woolly vest and a blue woolly vest — the former just looks warmer. Blue seems linked with loneliness and depression — when one is 'blue-devilled', has a 'fit of the blues', 'Blues' music, etc. Blue was worn by prostitutes and so we have 'blue', implying obscenity, cancelled out with a blue pencil (an association of the last World War). The German blau can also mean drunk, and it is claimed that alcohol causes visual images to become more blue and distant than normal.[1]

Even the warmer colours have their problem areas, although generally they are a little more positive. Apart from 'red for danger', one 'paints the town red', has a 'red-letter day', although 'sees red' when annoyed. But modern associations of the 'red cross' bring to mind help and assistance to victims of war and accident.

Yellow is often associated with cowardice and other undesirable attributes. Any one of these meanings could have sunk into our unconscious mind at an early age, to surface later as a 'dislike'.

If therefore you have a favourite colour, or find yourself always turning to one particular colour for dress or home surroundings, then the colour preference guide which follows may give you some insight into the reasons for this choice. Our colour preferences often change over the years and we may go through phases of wearing a particular colour, say blue, at a time when we very much desire peace and stability in our lives.

However, before you consult the colour list, please remember that these *are* only guidelines and nothing more. Whilst it seems that some persons with psychiatric problems do have violent love/hate reactions to colour, the majority of people tend not to be so extreme. If you do dislike a colour intensely, it might be interesting to find out why, but it doesn't mean that you're due for a session with the nearest psychiatrist!

White — symbolic of purity, innocence and naïvety. It has strong connotations of youth and freshness. A touch of white in the dress always looks fresh and attractive and on young girls white usually looks appealing and appropriate. Certain religious groups wear white, to symbolize purity of heart and a desire for simplicity or the simple life but when it is worn continuously for reasons other than religious convictions, and by rather older folk, it may suggest someone who is rather immature, someone with a desire for perfection and with impossible ideals, maybe someone who is vainly trying to recapture their lost youth and freshness. But worn in conjunction with other colours it shows a lively and well-balanced personality. We all need a touch of white in our lives.

Red — this is the colour of strength, health and vitality. It is often the colour chosen by someone outgoing, aggressive, vigorous and impulsive — or who would like to be! It goes with an ambitious nature but those who choose it can be abrupt and crude at times, determined to get all they can out of life. They may be quick to judge people and take sides. They are usually optimistic and can't stand monotony, being rather restless and expecting to be riding high all the time. They are not usually very introspective folk and therefore not too aware of their own shortcomings. They find it hard to be objective and tend to blame others for any mishaps. If an outwardly quiet person is very fond of red, they either feel the need for the warmth, strength and life-giving qualities of red, or blanket their true feelings under a sober exterior. Generally though it is chosen by those with open and uncomplicated natures, with a sympathy and zest for life.

As with any other colour, too much red is the sign of imbalance and if you are an introspective person given to red, it might be as well to ask yourself why you need it so much.

Maroon — Birren's interpretation of maroon is 'passion tempered by conscience or adversity'. In short, harsh experience has probably matured one into a likeable and generous person. It is a favourite with those who have been somewhat battered by life but have come through. It indicates a well disciplined 'red' personality — one who has had difficult experiences and has not come through unmarked, but who has grown and matured in the process.

Pink — embodies the gentler qualities of red. It symbolizes love and affection without passion and in women, tends to be linked with maternal types. Someone very fond of pink desires protection, special treatment and a sheltered life. They require affection, and like to feel loved and secure. The implications of red may be frightening for them and often the 'baby pink' worn by sometimes rather large ladies may reveal a desire to be looked upon as delicate and fragile. However it is a colour with warm connotations and those for whom it is the favourite tend to be charming and gentle, if a trifle indefinite.

Pink comes in a variety of tints from a rich strawberry to a pale apple-blossom and looks lovely as a secondary in your colour schemes but too much of it does rather give the impression that one is living in a cloud-cuckoo land where everything is seen through 'rose-coloured' spectacles.

Orange — the colour of luxury and pleasure which appeals to the flamboyant and fun-loving, who like a lively social round. They may be inclined to dramatize a bit, and people notice them, but they are generally good-natured and popular. They don't however care for someone else hogging the limelight and may get a trifle sulky if this goes on for too long! They can be superficial, fickle and vacillating but on the whole they like people and have a 'hail-fellow-well-met' attitude and a distinct gift of the gab. While they try hard to be agreeable, they tend not to notice the slings and arrows of misfortune, especially other people's! According to Harold Bopst[2] orange is the colour of youth, strength, fearlessness, curiosity and restlessness. It adds stimulus to cool colours and its complementary is blue.

Orange is one of those colours we can all do with a little of, and it adds an invigorating touch to an otherwise dull colour scheme. Overall it can be rather too much, although diluted down as apricot, for example, it has enough of pink in it to curb its more exuberant qualities. In the unlikely event of someone wanting to surround themselves with orange, or always wearing it, one would think they felt a great need for the stimulating qualities of both red and yellow.

Yellow — another of the primaries and fairly popular. It is the colour of happiness, wisdom and imagination. A strong liking for yellow reveals the mentally adventurous, searching for novelty and self-fulfilment. Among their ranks are the high-minded and philosophic, especially drawn to cults and pantheistic and occult organizations. It also usually goes with a sunny and shrewd personality, with a good business head and a strong sense of humour. It is the colour of intellectuality and all things to do with the mind. 'Yellow' people are usually clear and precise thinkers who have a good opinion of their own mental capabilities and who have lofty ideals. They do at times tend to shun responsibility, preferring freedom of thought and action. They also like admiration but angle for it more subtly than red or orange. Being another warm colour like red, yellow has some similar attributes but on a mental level, whereas red tends to be on the physical, but both share qualities such as impatience, a mentally outgoing attitude (though not so much physically for yellow — in fact they may be rather shy). They usually have strong convictions and can be rather stubborn and opinionated.

Yellow does have a strongly negative side and when overdone can be unpleasant. But for something or someone that needs brightening up, a dark room or a boring item of clothing, yellow in all its .various applications brings in a touch of sunshine and good cheer. Not liking yellow may well point to a fear of introspection, of dipping too deeply into one's own mental depths, or of being caught up in ideas that may cause one to feel trapped or forever allied to some uncomfortable thoughts. So many people are afraid of being alone with their own thoughts, or of breaking away from the conventional, or being caught up in the swirling waters of the mind — a touch of yellow would do them good, and throw a bright beam of light onto hitherto unexplored regions of themselves. Its complementary colour is violet.

Green — the colour of harmony and balance. It symbolizes hope, renewal and peace, and is usually liked by the gentle and sincere. They are generally frank, community-minded people, with a moral, but not prudish approach to life. They are usually fairly sociable but really prefer the quiet and peace of a country life and in fact sometimes prefer peace at any price, with all its negative connotations. They can be too self-effacing, modest and patient and so often get exploited by others. Usually refined, civilized and reputable — but they do tend to do the popular thing rather too often. They are often very good teachers, if a trifle garrulous.

Green can sometimes be a very depressing colour and too much gives a cool and detached impression. If you find yourself continually picking out clothes in green, or always surrounding yourself with it, it may be that you suffer from quite a high level of anxiety of which you are quite unaware. Green gives that feeling of everything being right in the world — the permanence and harmony of nature in an insecure and hostile environment. If you overdo it, it may be time to find out if your anxieties can be reduced and to reorganize your life upon more relaxed lines. In dress and home, try to liven up green with warmer colours in all their tints and shades — red being its complementary something along these lines would be suitable, rather than yellow, which does not show either colour to advantage.

Blue — usually regarded as everyone's favourite colour, along with red. One can sink into it peacefully, feel gentled by its qualities of compassion and caring, all 'mother' qualities, feminine, soft and soothing. It is a retreat from the harsh, unkind world of everyday life. However, it is also the colour of deliberation and introspection, conservatism and duty. Blue people can be rigid and self-righteous — they think their intentions are honest but they sometimes manipulate reason for their own ends. 'Blues' like to be part of a group, where for example 'reds' have an individual and bold approach to life. Sensitive and self-controlled blue likes to be admired for steady character, wisdom and sagacity — although this is really not always apparent! Blue is a good mixer, affectionate and faithful, perhaps even sentimental, but not one of life's pioneers, being cautious in word, action and dress. They often have fixed and inflexible beliefs and are sometimes worriers — especially about what others think. Blue might be said to epitomize the down-to-earth (but not in the red sense) character who has no time for something he can't understand. Blue also has a talent for self-justification and this is where the self-righteous side comes into play. They are however sociable folk and loyal friends, if somewhat suspicious of strangers, especially flamboyant ones! They do rather feel that everyone should lead an upright and sober life like themselves — at least outwardly! Being patient and persevering, they are likely to do well and make good students. They will be conscientious (usually) in their work but not inspired.

It doesn't sound as if blue is one of those colours that should be anyone's favourite, does it? But like all the others, it has its positive and negative aspect and the world would be a very sorry place without the blue of sea and sky, of flowers and streams. It is the colour of the cloak of the Virgin Mary, the Mother Goddess, symbolic of all the positive feminine qualities. Excitable 'red' people sometimes prefer blue because of its promising attributes of peace and equanimity. While weak persons crave strength the strong often seek gentleness and kindness to complement their own lack in this regard. Relief can be found through blue although the extrovert who prefers blue will show himself in his 'true colours' before long. Its complementary colour is orange and other qualities linked with it are serenity, dignity, spaciousness, sobriety, rest and peace.

If you find yourself choosing blue rather too often, it could mean that you want to bury your head in the sand, as it were, sink into the oblivion of blue and forget the trials and tribulations of your life. A continual desire for peace and oblivion points to some problem or conflict in the life, as most of us like a little excitement now and then. If at all possible 'blues' should make an effort to be more open-minded and flexible. That nasty outside world may not be as bad as you think — try a touch of orange to brighten yourself up!

Blue-Green — this is an attractive but strange mix from the point of view of colour preferences. Both Birren and Luscher and other researchers seem to think of it as basically a colour chosen by people with a high opinion of themselves, exacting and discriminating — even fussy! They are often poised and attractive persons who inspire envy and annoyance in those who feel less well endowed. It can be a sign of those who take love rather than give it. Sensitive, intellectual and refined, with an outer confidence and sophistication, blue-greens are also persevering, stable but rather detached. They are generally very capable and tend to reject help or guidance. It seems a rather 'Aquarian' colour — its subjects always willing to help others but in a rather detached manner. They have excellent taste, are courteous and charming, but expect admiration, favour and respect and take these for granted.

Those choosing **Turquoise** are similarly complex, imaginative and original. They often drive themselves hard and there is occasionally quite a state of turmoil under that outwardly cool exterior.

Lavender — an offshoot of purple, is a pretty colour but somehow too much of it can be rather cool and offputting. It is associated with vanity, ultra-femininity and aloofness and is often chosen by the sort of person who 'lives on a higher plane,' who never notices anything sordid and who is always impeccable and beautifully dressed. They are on a continual quest for culture and the refined things of life, high and noble causes — provided their hands don't get dirty and nothing 'earthy' is involved. All in all, perhaps a bit 'twee' but you can depend on them to be charming, witty and civilized and endowed with all the social graces. They are usually artistic (or have pretensions that way) and like to cultivate others on the same uplifted plane, and are very impressed by greatness. There is often great determination to get one's own way. Mauve and lavender people are inclined to live in a world of fantasy but there's a commonsense streak hidden away together with a very strong instinct of self-survival! There is often great creative talent, especially in design of various kinds — one thinks of the rather exotic male dress-designer, or the hostess who holds elegant little parties where all the guests are very refined and cultivated.

It may be chosen by people who desire to get away from

sordid conditions in their life, or who have higher aspirations than those present in their life style. Its complementary would be one of the variations of yellow.

Purple — now here's a really flamboyant colour although it is not all that popular. It has connotations of mourning, solemnity, pomp and ceremony. It is certainly not an easy colour to live with in large quantities, being very 'heavy' and needing a powerful personality to carry it off well. If you really prefer purple to all other colours you may be suffering from delusions of grandeur — or maybe you really **are** grand! At the least it shows a strong desire to be individual — even eccentric! It is a colour usually associated with the Madame Arcarti type of clairvoyant — all beads and purple plush robes. Purple people are usually fastidious, witty and sensitive, but with a strong desire to be 'different.' They have Jupiterian attributes, being expansive and extrovert, but also highly-strung, temperamental and 'artistic.' They can also be aloof, sarcastic and introspective when 'misunderstood.' More interested in culture than humanity, purples often have high-falutin ideas about life. On the good side they are unconventional and tolerant, interested in philosophy and often very verbose about their ideals while not actually doing anything about them! They are dignified and like to achieve a position of authority, which they regard as their natural place. They can be intellectual snobs. Bopst considers purple the colour of the nucleus of all life impulses — the colour of the opening bud, the first streak of dawn and the last ray of the setting sun. He maintains that purple can produce a high state of exhilaration, but this is soon followed by an equally intense state of irritation, and finally depression. He quotes the analogy of hearing a single pleasing sound; however pleasing in itself it cannot be endured for long.

If purple is really your colour maybe you should get down from that throne once in a while and brighten up your colour scheme with some variations of its complementary, yellowy-green.

Brown — we come down to earth with a bump when considering brown — the colour for solid and substantial people, the world's workers, with stamina and patience. They are usually very conscientious, dutiful, dependable, steady and conservative. The brain may be a bit slow but gets there in the end. Your real brown freaks are not impulsive creatures, and maybe a bit inarticulate and tactless. But they love responsibility and can always be relied on to do that job that nobody else wants and thus other people take advantage of them. They are salt-of-the-earth types and are usually kindly except when they come up against the world's loafers. Browns can be rather careful about their finances and don't believe in throwing good money after bad. 'Meanness' might be an exaggeration but it has been known. They can be very obstinate in habits and convictions and don't like change. The less-brown natives are sometimes shy but warm-hearted, liking to feel needed, which seems to result in them always helping the underdog. They know how to strike a good bargain but don't believe in making strenuous efforts of a physical or mental nature. Their real problem is inflexibility and inability to adapt easily.

Overdoing brown, of course, means overdoing the more negative side of brown — being too plodding, dull and inert. But brown is a very good background colour which can be brightened up by more colourful accessories. It can act as a ballast, balancing out an otherwise too exotic colour scheme.

If you find yourself always wearing brown, other than for reasons of expediency, then try to break away occasionally, or brighten it up with cheerful accessories — it seems to go well with most other colours especially something unusual like pink, turquoise or apricot.

Grey — this is the colour of caution and compromise, a balance between the extremes of black and white, a search for composure and peace without expending any inner sources of energy. Those who like grey turn away from excitement and worldly things, thus it is often a colour worn by the dedicated, who will work hard without reward. It is often preferred by older people who like life to run on an even keel with few ups and downs but when worn continually by someone young, suggests a withdrawal from life, a renunciation of all the good things abounding in the world and a blurring of insight, a suppression of the personality. Often greys have business ability and tend to overwork. Like brown, it is a good background colour if livened up with warm and bright colours.

Black — the colour of mystery! It is often worn by those who wish to give this impression but for the truly sophisticated is dignified and impressive, without being too showy. When dark colours are always worn it can signify the suppression of inner desires and worldly aims, suggesting hidden depths and secret longings. It is much worn by women in male-dominated countries where it is presumably worn for 'protection' but one gains the impression that such women are encouraged to fix their minds on higher things, negate their personalities and simply exist to fill the role of wife and mother. Black can look magnificent or dowdy, depending on the wearer, but an all-black ensemble can be rather like the advertisement for 'Keep Death off the Road'!

Figure 2: Complementary Colours

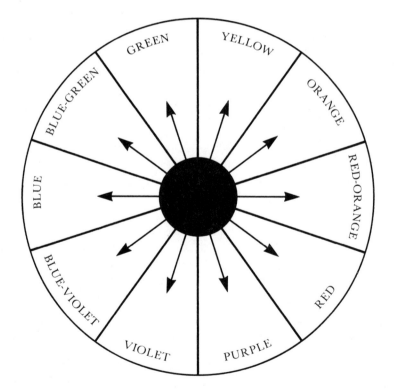

Colour and Psychology

Birren gives examples of the work of various psychologists such as Felix Deutsch, Kurt Goldstein and others too numerous to mention here.[3] From such studies it appears that to many mentally or emotionally disturbed people, especially schizophrenics, colour is an unwanted intrusion into their life, and they neither like it nor want it. On the other hand people suffering from exhaustion, or nervous breakdown, show little reaction to colour at all. Manic-depressives, however, delight in colour (presumably on 'good' days!). In the Rorschach Test (the inkblot tests in black and white and colour) it has been noted that introverted patients tend to reject colour.

It has been found that people with anxiety states tend to have a predilection for green, the 'red' impulses of hatred, aggression and sex being denied. Researcher Eric P. Moss[4] therefore finds it unsurprising that red is the choice of the manic and hypomanic patient 'giving the tumult of his emotions their "burning" and "bloody" expression'.

Yellow is the colour of schizophrenia — the colour of the morbid mind. Whenever we observe its accumulative appearance there is quite likely to be a deep-lying psychotic disturbance. Note the work of such artists as Van Gogh and Louis Wain (famous for his drawings of cats) which in their latter days when both were severely mentally ill, became significantly flame-like in colouring and appearance. The depressive person paints in sombre shades of dark red and black, while the manic, in his state of over-excitement, uses a lot of bright, bold colour with lots of swirls and agitated lines. Painting is often very therapeutic in such cases, allowing the patient to express his feelings without having to struggle with words.

Brown relates to paranoia and blue is also associated with schizophrenia along with yellow. Under stress persons who like blue may tend to see the environment connected with their problems in some drastic manner. But blue is allied with conscious control of emotions and is the colour of circumspection.

It does not follow, of course, that because we favour red, or green, or yellow, that we are suffering from any of the above conditions. But nevertheless red is usually chosen by extroverts and yellow by persons having an intellectual bent, although it is also associated with mental deficiency!

Green is often the choice of persons who are superficially intelligent, social, chatty and with big appetites! Continual choice of green suggests escape from anxiety, sanctuary in the untroubled greenness of nature.

Narcissism is revealed by a preference for blue-green. It may indicate fastidiousness, sensitiveness and discrimination. Such persons often have pronounced self-love and self-sufficiency and are difficult patients for the psychiatrist.

One of the most readable researchers on the psychological aspects of colour is Dr Max Lüscher. His book *The Lüscher Colour Test*[5] has been translated into English and is quite easy for the intelligent layman to grasp, precise instructions being given for assessing one's own personality as well as that of others. As with all these 'Methods', caution should be exercised, as they are not meant to be used as party games.

Dr Lüscher's method entails choosing eight colours in order of preference. The test is based on the arrangement of these eight and their relationship to each other. If one chooses honestly, it can be quite a blow to one's ego how some of these combinations work out in terms of personality assessment! As with all such tests, once you know roughly the 'correct' answers, it becomes rather difficult to be objective and not cheat!

Without giving away too much of the test, it is interesting to compare Dr Lüscher's findings with those of other researchers. I tend to find these tests a little negative at times because it seems that whatever you choose, you can't win. But as they were presumably first devised for people with problems, we must keep this in mind and not despair if our personalities are less than perfect.

His colour cards (in the book version) are not all true primaries — the red is orange-red; blue is dark-blue; the green has a lot of blue in it; the violet has a lot of red; and the brown is a rather unattractive shade. Yellow is the only true primary. As none of the colours is, to my mind, particularly attractive, possibly this ensures that the person choosing the cards is more honest! You can check these colour meanings against those given earlier and in many instances there certainly seems to be a correlation.

Red is assigned most of the qualities already outlined in earlier pages. It is 'impulse will-to-win and all forms of vitality and power from sexual potency to revolutionary transformation'. Thus a rejected red (placed in a negative position on the test layout) often signifies physical and nervous exhaustion with its accompanying loss of potency or sexual desire, or possible heart or other disorders. Those for whom red occupies a prominent place are seeking experience and fullness of life and often throw themselves into activities that can be over-exaggerated — but this will be mitigated or confirmed by the colour which accompanies red in the test. All in all, most researchers seem in agreement as to the qualities of red. Whoever places red in the 'rejected' position is already over stimulated to the point where such a colour irritates because of the intensity of his problems, which may appear insoluble or over-demanding. He thus throws out anything suggestive of further stress.

Blue is often put in a position where it compensates for rejected red. These two are often aligned where business anxieties and possible heart disease are present and in fact Dr Lüscher regards them as an excellent early warning sign. The blue thus represents complete calm and contemplation of this colour has a pacifying effect on the nervous system and as other researchers have found, blood-pressure, pulse and respiration are all reduced, although according to Birren this is only a temporary effect, the condition reverting back even more than originally. Dark blue also represents contentment and fulfilment, 'truth and trust, love and dedication, surrender and devotion, representing traditional and eternal values'. So when this colour is given priority there is a great need for rest and relaxation and the chance to recover. This person wants a calm and orderly existence, free from contention. When chosen for a position standing on its own, as it were, and not 'compensating' it implies 'quietness of spirit, calmness of manner...and integrity'.

However, when blue is rejected, this can indicate an anxiety over business and personal relationships probably due to too exacting standards of perfection being desired. There is the wish to sever ties because of this and in turn this causes restlessness and mental turmoil. It may become difficult to concentrate and even lead to disturbance of the nervous system. Sometimes red is put in a compensatory position suggesting that the sufferer will make dramatic efforts for emotional fulfilment, either perhaps in promiscuous behaviour or in some dangerous or adventurous activity such as mountain climbing or car racing — although I find it hard to believe that all such enthusiasts are compensating for some great lack in their emotional make-up.

Green is also sometimes chosen as a compensation for rejected blue, and this suggests a proud and rebellious demand for independence. The green in this test has more blue than yellow, thus becoming blue-green, and the colour of the ego. Therefore someone who puts this in a prominent position places a high value on the 'I', his own self-awareness and self-affirmation. So if this is your most-favoured colour it reveals, subject to its companion colours, a desire to increase self-assertiveness. You may have a somewhat idealized picture of yourself and expect others to recognize this also! Green is proud and unchanging and very aware of his ego. Loss of face for 'greens' often results in ulcers and digestive and stomach upsets. This colour does of course have a positive side as its adherents are often forced to find expression in a quest for better conditions, improved health and so on, and here we have the reformer. Unfortunately green does tend to moralize to others and put himself on a pedestal. Green likes to impress and would rather be admired than loved. But those who reject green and place it in a weak position also want these things but feel unable to achieve them and therefore suffer from a sense of pressure, sometimes exploding outwardly as a chest or heart complaint. Rejected green therefore means, according to to Lüscher, 'anxiety to liberate himself from the tensions imposed by non-recognition'. Extreme cases are those unhappy folk who are so stubborn and self-opinionated as to be their own worst enemies.

Blue is often chosen as compensation (that is, put in the place a healthy green would normally occupy) as effort is no longer required; red compensation reveals itself in loss of self-control and impatience. Green in a 'normal' position in the test is of course part of a natural urge we all have to express ourselves and be recognized by our fellows.

Yellow is the only true primary used in the test. It indicates qualities of expansiveness and relaxation. Although yellow also increases blood-pressure, pulse and respiration rates, it does not do so with the consistency of red. Yellow corresponds to sunlight, cheerfulness and happiness, but it has a somewhat unstable and uncertain quality... rather Mercurial, in fact. If yellow is first choice, it shows the desire for release and the hope of better things to come. When it occupies a major position there is not only a great desire to escape from present conditions but a desire for change for the sake of change. If, as Dr Lüscher says, green is 'persistence and tension', yellow is 'change and relaxation'.

If yellow is rejected, then hopes have been dashed with a resultant inner turmoil. This may result in irritability and depression, often hopelessness. Blue is sometimes chosen instead and shows a need to hang onto the familiar and safe. Or, if green is chosen, there may be efforts to compensate by striving after prestige and position. Unhappy 'yellow' can have problems with the sympathetic and parasympathetic nervous systems. Yellow is usually preferred by people of an intellectual bent — but it is as well to remember that it is also associated with mental deficiency! Its rejection may be indicative of a dislike of probing too deeply into one's own mental processes and inner feelings.

Violet — a very red-blue mix, that tends to fall into the category mentioned in the previous list of colours — that of the fantasy world. The person who puts this particular violet in a prominent place wants magic and glamour for himself as well as others. While this may indicate some immaturity, the world would be a duller place if there were no 'violet' people. But there is a quality of unreality and wish fulfilment in the make-up of those whose main choice this is and it is often chosen by the naïve and unsophisticated. Glandular and hormonal activity during pregnancy may result in a temporary preference for violet and this also sometimes applies to people with a thyroid problem. Again to those suffering from emotional insecurity, violet suggests a magical world where everything comes right in the end. The true 'violet' type is sensitive and charming, often casts a spell over themselves and others, but does not want responsibility.

Brown — this is a dark yellow-red. Those who choose it for a major position are emphasizing the body's sensory condition. Brown indicates physical sensation and depending where it is placed, can reveal a degree of physical discomfort. The rootless and homeless often make brown their first choice as it suggests security and ease, and a place of one's own. It can indicate a need for physical ease, or release from some painful or uncomfortable condition such as illness, or a state of conflict and unsolvable problems. When brown is rejected, physical comfort is seen as a weakness — this reveals the 'cold baths and hair shirt' type of person. But when the body is denied in one way it will retaliate in another, probably with some form of compulsive behaviour. One is reminded of some of the early saints who were always battling with unseemly visions! In a normal position brown simply reveals the average person's desire for reasonable comfort, home and security.

Grey — is the most neutral colour of all, neither dark nor light. It represents a sort of no-man's land, an area of separation between two zones. Chosen in first place it indicates that the chooser wants to wall everything off and be uncommitted and uninvolved in anything. Whatever colour follows usually points to an unadmitted desire represented by that choice.

Grey is however part of our normal make-up and those who reject it in an equally strong fashion may try to involve themselves in too much, becoming tiresome meddlers who are anxious to miss nothing. Grey boxed in by two colours reveals a desire only to experience through the qualities of the first and to block off the second.

Grey in a prominent place in the test suggests self-deception and can be descriptive of people who are often powerful in business and industry, another urge which psychologists consider may be due to a desire to escape from some unwarrantable anxiety!

Black — expresses the idea of nothingness and extinction, renunciation and surrender. Whoever chooses black as first choice wants to renounce everything as a protest against existing conditions. If for instance, red follows, then exaggerated desires may compensate for all that is deficient; if blue, then complete tranquillity and harmony are expected to restore things to rights; if yellow, then some sudden change of course — or a miracle — is expected to end one's troubles. In the 'normal' position it indicates the usual human desire not to have to relinquish anything and to be in control of one's life.

From the above it will be seen that there are many tie-ups

between Dr Lüscher's findings and those of other researchers and the intriguing question is why certain colours correspond as they do to certain characteristics in our personalities. To answer this we can only return to the first chapter where in the comparatively short history of mankind colours and their associations were firmly imprinted upon the collective mind: red — heat, blood, life and danger; blue — sky, heaven, peace, mother; green — growth (and decay); yellow — sun, warmth, happiness; white — purity, cleanliness, perfection; black — mystery, death, and annihilation. Many more subtle colours and qualities have arisen since those early days but they all stem from the basic primaries.

Most normal people use a mixture of colours for personal use but as all of us have a few quirks here and there in our personalities, it might be a useful exercise to investigate these. Here such tests as the above may be helpful, although what seems to be forgotten is the fact that most of us would never do anything if it were not for hidden urges and inner stresses, driving us to take some drastic action. It is only when these stresses become unbearable or when we can see no way out, that these tests are truly valuable.

References

1. H. Rossotti, *Colour: Why the World Isn't Grey* (Pelican
2. Harold Bopst, *Colour and Personality* (USA)
3. Faber Birren, *Color and the Human Response* (Van Nostrand Reinhold Co. Inc., 1978)
4. Faber Birren, *Light, Color and the Environment* (Van Nostrand Reinhold Co. Inc., 1969).
5. *The Lüscher Colour Test*, trans. by Ian Scott (Jonathan Cape Ltd., London, 1970)

4.
Colour In Our Being

Whether the aura actually exists or not is still a matter of controversy between those who claim to see it and measure it and those who can't. However, for the purposes of this chapter it will be simpler to assume that it exists and for those unhappy with this assumption a perusal of the works of Professor Harold Saxton Burr and Dr J. Kilner is recommended.

The aura (from the Greek word *avra* meaning 'breeze') is not a modern phenomenon dreamed up by 'psychics and 'mystics'. Our ancestors knew all about auras and from very early times artists have depicted them around the heads of saints and other holy persons. It was hardly likely that such a thought would have arisen without some basis in fact. Words such as halo, nimbus, aureole, and glory are descriptive of various parts of the aura — a 'glory' for instance, is described as 'a circle of rays surrounding the head of a saint' and an aureole is the radiance surrounding the entire body.

People of psychic sensitivity have often described a radiance surrounding not only saintly persons but also ordinary folk as well. In the Bible, for example, Moses' face, when he came down from the mountain, 'shone so that they were afraid to come nigh him'.[1]

Not only human beings, but every creature and everything in nature appears to be surrounded by a radiance, ranging from the faint hazy outline to be seen around a stone to the rather larger aura of a tree. We know that every living thing gives off various electrical and other emanations — we can't generally see them but they can be sensed and recorded by delicate instruments as well as by sensitive people — in fact people are far more sensitive than any instrument. If we could see ourselves for the swirling mass of atoms that we are, it would be very difficult for us to regard ourselves as 'solid bodies' thereafter.

Since the advent of Kirlian photography there has been a great deal more interest shown in the aura and unfortunately many people have made the mistake of equating this with the 'rays' shown in the photographs. While they are somewhat similar in appearance to auric rays, it is probable that they have more of a link with electrical emanations from the body but they are certainly not the same thing as the human aura, unless possibly one regards them as that part of it nearest to the physical body. The aura itself is much larger and more finely constituted. It can nevertheless be seen and felt by those who are sensitive enough to do so. Most people can, after a little practice, see the basic auric outline, but anything further than that usually requires some degree of clairvoyant sight.

To catch a glimpse of the average aura can be difficult unless there is something noteworthy about it. Auras vary considerably in density and structure and even those who can normally see them are not always able to do so. That part of the aura closest to the physical body manifests itself as a narrow band of 'transparent' light, sometimes a misty white, about a half inch wide. From this the aura can expand to anything from two feet wide or even much larger, depending on the individual. Within this auric body can be seen the fluctuating colours which give it its identity.

For basic purposes, the aura of humans can be divided into three separate parts, corresponding to the basic 'bodies' which reside in and around the physical vehicle. These comprise the Etheric, or Vital body — that closest to the physical, which is said to leave the body in sleep or unconsciousness; next comes the Astral (this term can be confusing as it sometimes refers to the Etheric — depending on your school of thought) — the Emotional body — that which supplies most of the auric colouring; and the third is the Mental body — that of the intellect and all its attributes. The aura of women is usually seen more easily than that of men, which may be due to them having more developed emotional bodies and to their being more at ease in this mode of expression than men, who tend to pride themselves on being rationalistic, thinking individuals, thus restricting their emotional expression. Beyond these three levels there are even more subtle 'bodies' of varying degrees of spirituality and their colours are usually only briefly glimpsed.

To 'see' an aura is to some extent an acquired knack which is easier than people think and you may have been aware of them for years without realizing it. The first essential is to be relaxed. Look slightly above and beyond the head of your subject, gazing into infinity. Don't try too hard or it will just elude you. A neutral background with no distracting colours is best, although some people prefer a dark background. Stand your subject against a plain door or curtain and be at least ten feet away from them. Even against a coloured background the colours will sometimes be strong enough to override it. You can practice with non-humans — animals, plants and trees. You may not succeed for some time but most people, after a while, are able to see the faint band of mist closest to the physical body.

Naturally there are various pitfalls to avoid if 'looking' in this way — the most obvious being that of visual aberration. Our eyes play many tricks upon us and we have to be very honest with ourselves as to what we think we are seeing. One of the main problems is that of eye fatigue. When the eyes become tired they tend to 'see' a bluish-green haze around the object of vision — you can experiment and see if this happens in your case. Similarly, complementary colour effects can be misleading — someone wearing bright red will appear to have a green aura; likewise if they are wearing a blue hat or have orange hair, the complementary colour will comprise the 'aura'. Only practice, and comparing notes with other sensitives will give you the experience and confidence that what you are seeing is definitely the aura. Get acquainted with some of the tricks your eyes can play and then you should be able to sort the wheat from the chaff.

However, do not lose heart if you cannot see anything — there is a way of sensing auric colours and that is by mentally tuning into your subject. But it is best to begin with a practical exercise. Engage the help of a co-operative friend and seat them in a chair. Then hold your hands a few inches away from your friend's head and try to sense any radiations within this area. You will first become conscious of waves of bodily warmth — the head gives off quite a bit of heat. Then perhaps if your friend is tense and unrelaxed you will begin to sense this as a kind of vibration coming from them. Slowly withdraw your hands until you reach a point where this tension appears to cease — this could be the limits of the 'astral' body aura, at least. You should try to remain in a relaxed state yourself during this procedure and if so, you can then focus your mind upon the thought of auric colours, waiting to see if any specific colours relating to the subject appear in your mind. This is rather more difficult and takes some practice. Later, you should be able to look at a person, mentally tune in and receive a colour impression of their aura. This is not telepathy, or trying to pick up their thoughts — it is a procedure which we all unconsciously use during our daily life, a continual assessment of those around us. Test the auras of as many different people as you can and you will begin to get a general idea of how much they can vary in breadth and density. Some will feel 'all over the place' and very thin or diffuse; others will be too tight, compact and withdrawn; but the majority of people will have a fairly normal aura of between eighteen inches and two feet in depth, surrounding their head and body in a generally ovoid shape. 'Cold spots' or unusual emanations in the aura can be signs of damage or breaks and these will be dealt with in a later chapter. The aura is a very important protective mechanism which must be treated with the same respect as one treats the physical body.

Our auras fulfil a very important task — that of protecting us from a variety of subtle and not-so-subtle energies, emanations from various sources, thought-forms, disease organisms, and minor bumps and bruises, in much the same way that the physical skin protects the inner organs, and skeleton structure of the body. In shamanistic teachings, such as those described in the books of Carlos Castenada and Max Freedom Long the auric field is described as a mass of fine fibres standing out at right angles to the body. Depending on one's state of health and personal power, these fibres can be extended indefinitely, especially from the solar plexus and other chakric areas, for purposes of telepathic contact, telekinesis (moving objects without any apparent means of doing so), clairvoyance and most other paranormal abilities. In some cases of poltergeist activity no doubt the instigator is unconsciously using personal energy through the medium of the auric rays. A ray, or fibre, can be extended to an object, or another person, for any variety of reasons. A good example of the auric energy being used for personal objectives is in one of Carlos Castenada's books[2] where the shaman Genaro manages to attach himself to rocks overhanging a waterfall by means of auric 'fibres'. He is then

able to take incredible leaps from rock to rock by these
'tentacles' which keep him in place as securely as a fly on the
ceiling.

It is also possible, in a more modest way, to divine the
strength or weakness of people's auras — there is a distinct
'resistance' when one comes up against a very strong auric
field. Large and formidable people have an aura one can almost
bounce off! It is no wonder that kings were always credited with
so much personal power when you think of someone like Henry
VIII — who besides being physically large, had the authority of
kingship behind him, giving a double boost to a no doubt
powerful personality. There is the story of the Egyptian king
who accidentally touched one of his courtiers with his staff. The
poor man was convinced he would die on the spot because of the
royal power; however Pharaoh was concerned and spoke kindly
to him, thus restoring him to normal.

We are making auric contacts all the time — some very
minor but others forming very strong bonds indeed. Not all of
these are beneficial of course, but are nevertheless there just the
same. We constantly monitor other people's auras and they
our's and some we do not care for and withdraw protectively
into our own shell. Others we respond to, and feel in harmony
with and we are drawn automatically to such persons.

It is very important that the auric field be as strong as we can
make it. How to do this will be more fully described in the last
chapter, but basically it is simply a matter of thinking about it
and trying to imagine it surrounding the body rather like a
protective force-field around a spacecraft, or an atmosphere
around a planet. The more one thinks about it in this manner,
the stronger it becomes. There are of course the apocryphal
stories of adepts with such strong auras that bullets bounce off
them!

Really gifted clairvoyants can study an individual's aura to
the extent that they can diagnose illness and winkle out one's
character secrets. To such people we are going about with our
lights 'full on', as easily readable as a book. Fortunately for our
peace of mind there are not too many able to 'see' to this extent
but even if you never succeed in seeing or sensing colours you
can gain a general impression of the state of a particular aura.
There seems to be a brightness around some people; a dark
cloud around others. Mostly we register these impressions
without really thinking about them. Next time you do feel

something of this sort, try to analyse exactly what gives this impression — is it the facial expression, the stance of the physical form, or something beyond them both?

From Paracelsus to Mesmer, and from Mesmer to the present day, many persons of scientific and intellectual bent have endeavoured to investigate the aura. One of the most widely quoted is Dr J. Kilner, Medical Electrician at St Thomas's Hospital, London. In his book *The Human Atmosphere* he described a method involving a glass screen incorporating a cyanine dye, through which the human aura could be perceived. He maintained that every human body was surrounded by an emanation extending some eighteen inches to two feet in all directions, ovoid in shape. This varied slightly from day to day and became rather more difficult to see during illness. Dr Kilner, in the revised version of the book, *The Human Aura*, seemed of the opinion that the aura one was dealing with was an ultraviolet phenomenon. He noted that some women had the ability to change their auric colours at will. His book describes in great detail the diagnosis of auric fields in humans, although it was mostly ignored by the medical profession. Many clairvoyants also dispute that the aura can actually be seen through Kilner screens, maintaining that you have to be clairvoyant anyway to be able to see it and that therefore Dr Kilner must have been clairvoyant himself. It is a fact that not everyone can see an aura when looking through Kilner screens and they may well be just a psychological prop.

Kilner goggles are still available for those who wish to experiment with his methods although it is preferable to try to see the aura without such aids. Further work in this field has been carried on by Henry Boddington, who actually devised the goggles and fitted them with double glasses between which the dye solution could be placed. Dr Kilner was able to diagnose ailments and injuries by his method of auric viewing in much the same way as diagnoses are made from Kirlian photography nowadays[3] and possibly here again some degree of clairvoyance is involved.

Whatever your method of registering auric colours, the following notes may give you some hints on diagnosis. This is again a very individual matter and should only be regarded as a guide. You will find that you will require to modify or adapt some of these interpretations according to your own findings. But on a very general basis they provide a fairly accurate framework. The main colours of the aura are those of the rainbow and here they overlap at times with colour interpretation in other fields.

Many colour therapists work in accordance with the 'vibratory rays of the universe' and S.J.J.Ouseley in his informative little book *Science of the Aura*[4] interprets the seven colour rays as follows:

> Violet — spiritual power
> Indigo — intuition
> Blue — inspiration
> Green — energy
> Yellow — wisdom
> Orange — health
> Red — life

Here we can see the extent to which they fit in with colour interpretations in earlier chapters. However it is a rather too general assessment for auric diagnosis but it is nevertheless a useful guide.

Let us commence at the most physical level — the colour of life. To the finer sight there will be many graduations of hue, in varying degrees of clarity: these are interpreted through experience and in fact may take many years of practice to achieve.

Red in the aura, if clear and bright, reveals an abundance of vitality, sexual power, and an active, outgoing, generous and possibly materialistic nature. Red is usually not the main colour, and may only appear temporarily, depending on the mood of the subject and whether they are in some state of excitation, such as anger, desire, etc. A muddy or dark red denotes negative emotions such as hate, malice and other destructive passions. Combined with black it suggests very unpleasant characteristics. If one loses one's temper, one imagines red sparks coming out of one's head — this can be literally seen at such times by the visually sensitive, but is only a temporary effect which can however cause the head aura to open, resulting in a headache or feeling of depletion. But a healthy red now and then, as with everything else, means that we are alive and kicking.

Blue-reds and orange-reds are obviously diluted reds and correspondingly affected by their companion colour. A lovely rosy pink is usually associated with unselfish love, while the presence of dull brownish grey could indicate that selfishness of some kind has crept in. There are subtler variations of red but interpretation of these best comes with experience and not many are able to tune in so finely.

Orange is also regarded as a rather worldly and materialistic colour to have in the aura, but again it depends on the actual hue or shade. A muddy orange can indicate selfishness, an urge 'to get there first', pride and obstinacy. But a clear orange, while of a material quality, shows normal ambition and perhaps denotes the down-to-earth person with little time for the fantastic. A pleasing apricot blends orange and pink for the kindly, commonsensical, well-balanced type of person. Again it is a sign of energy — physical vitality combined with intellectual activity (red and yellow) — but if dominating the aura, leaves out the softening qualities of blue and pink. Dominant orange is usually the sign of an ambitious, worldly sort of person, usually fairly healthy and not given to too much introspection.

Yellow represents mental activity and can be noted in most auras when the subject is concentrating, reading or writing, or engaged in any other left brain activity. Unless one is of the predominantly 'thinker' type of person, it tends to come and go. A good yellow is an excellent colour to have in the aura and it sometimes brightens into gold if the person's thinking is on a highly spiritual level. Maybe next time the vicar gives a particularly good sermon it might be worthwhile taking a look at his aura! Dingy yellows are suspect — often indicating suspicion and jealously, clouded thinking, or at least aimless dreaming. Good yellow aura people are usually bright and cheerful, capable and resourceful, but as said, yellow appears in most auras from time to time.

Green, with the exception of the darker shades, is usually a good colour to have in the aura, but as it is the 'energy' colour it can also indicate depletion. I remember an occasion when a friend was giving a talk and several people present who normally 'never saw anything' noted a brightish green aura around her. Normally this lady had a brilliantly coloured aura with pink, yellow and blue intermingling, so the contrast was extreme. She had on this occasion just recovered from 'flu and her energy level was very low.

Some sensitives consider that a light green in the aura denotes healing ability. Other schools of thought hold that mid-green indicates adaptability and versatility (though this depends on your personal interpretation of 'mid-green'); clear green, sympathy; while the darker shades suggest treachery and deceit. Too much green, as in other areas, can give a rather negative feeling of detachment and non-commitment. Green and blue combined, to my mind, always indicates intuition or at least great sensitivity.

Blue. There are many aspects of blue and nearly all are indicative of positive qualities — integrity, sincerity, a strong sense of the religious, inspiration, compassion and kindliness. As the intensity of blue deepens so the above-mentioned qualities are enhanced. Indigo, for instance, is said to show a high degree of spirituality, while paler hues suggest such qualities as self-reliance and idealism. Most people's auras have a fair amount of blue in them and while its absence does not of course mean that they do not manifest any of the above qualities, it probably indicates that they are on a more mental or physical level, according to whether the predominant colour is yellow or red. The 'true-blue' personality is usually emotionally well-developed and more of a 'feeling' type of individual. Again, muddied colours of any sort indicate a lessening of the positive qualities, a clouding and disruption of their true function.

Violet. This is the colour of cosmic-consciousness, the colour that indicates the free-ranging mind able to consider life and the universe without dogmatism, taking past and future in its scope, with an awareness that life is eternal and forever evolving.

This colour is rarely seen to dominate an aura and is usually only noted in the outer fringes, being an extension of the more spiritual auric bodies. Many New Age people have this colour in their auras, thus reflecting the awareness and idealism of the coming Aquarian epoch.

Grey. One can sometimes see all-grey auras and it doesn't necessarily mean the subject is depressed. But certainly it doesn't denote very exciting qualities for those who have it in their auras and they are likely to be very conventional, formal, and rather unadventurous, to say the least. It does indicate lack of imagination, although such people are often very good organizers. They are persistent and plodding and often described as 'loners' or 'oddballs'. Darker shades of grey can be attributed to severe depression or at least a very negative attitude towards life. Maybe we all get a bit grey at times but it shouldn't be a permanent state.

Black. Not a good colour at all to have in the aura. Any auras showing quantities of black should be regarded as having extremely negative aspects. Fortunately the truly 'black' aura is very rare, most people having some redeeming quality to their personalities. However if it does appear in combination with another colour, then that colour will indicate the direction of the specific negative quality in question. If mixed with red, for instance, which is the worst possible combination, it indicates hatred, cruelty and the basest of evil desires. Such people are too dangerous to get involved with and on such an occasion it might be advisable not to stop and examine their auras too closely, but get out while the going's good! A black and yellow aura would indicate an evil genius of the 'thinking' variety. Even so, such people may have redeeming qualities, being able to justify their evil acts to themselves on a purely mental level. After all, even some of the Nazi war criminals were known to have been affectionate fathers and husbands. A black and green aura could indicate treachery, envy of the worst kind, avarice — or possibly some severe health problem. A blackness in a specific part of the aura often points to a physical disorder of some nature, or can indicate an 'entity' or 'thought form' caught up in the auric field. Any blackness at all in the aura of a living person, or an entity from some other level of being, is to be regarded with extreme caution.

Silver is considered a mercurial and rather volatile colour in the aura and is usually associated with lively but rather unreliable people who perhaps have streaks of brilliance now and then. This colour generally emanates from the 'mental' body and therefore has all the detachment and superficiality that this might imply. It can sometimes be associated with excessive refinement of mind and attitudes — the 'higher plane' dwellers who tend to be a bit difficult to live up to.

Pink is a lovely colour to have in the aura, denoting love and affection, kindness and gentleness. Too much may indicate the 'rose-coloured spectacles' type of person, but they are usually warm and responsive people who are rarely aggressive or overwhelming in any way. A fair leavening of pink in the aura makes up for a lot of deficiencies and shows a nice balance when mixed with any of the other positive colours.

Brown. Touches of brown in the aura are said to indicate a very down-to-earth attitude, an aptitude for organization and a materialistic approach to life. It is the colour of the conventional, closed mind, with little emotion but a desire to dominate. It is not a happy colour to have in large amounts but the typical 'brown' aura would probably be so withdrawn and uptight that it would be rather difficult to see it anyway.

White. This is an interesting colour to have in the aura, although again this is subject to personal interpretation. In the experience of my own particular 'school' white in the aura has come to be regarded as a very useful indication of the type of person who is a 'transmitter' rather than a 'receiver'. Such persons would succeed in sending out telepathic impressions, healing thoughts, and possibly have the ability to manipulate various levels of energy rather than be manipulated by them. It suggests a 'positive' type of mind not too influenced by outside impressions. Medical people, exorcists, teachers of various kinds, and all who have to deal with situations where a detached but compassionate attitude is necessary, probably tend to have a certain amount of white in their auras. Mixed with the blue-green of intuition as well it would make for a formidable personality (in the psychic sense) who could combine all these qualities, receiving impressions on an emotional level but well able to evaluate them without getting too involved, and furthermore, to coolly formulate a solution and apply this in a positive and directive manner. White often indicates a good supply of psychic energy which can be utilized in the abovementioned way.

It must be remembered that the aura is constantly fluctuating according to our moods and emotions — as also it reflects our state of health on a physical level. It is our own personal aurora and reacts constantly to outside stimuli, much in the way that the earth's aurora is affected by particle streams from the sun, solar winds, and distant stars and planets. Unpleasant noise affects it very adversely, causing it constantly to flicker. However, if one is sufficiently relaxed, even a road-drill can be regarded with equilibrium! But sudden and severe shocks of various kinds can cause the aura to expand, become displaced or even 'break' in places, leaving the possessor unprotected and at the mercy of whatever happens to be passing at the time. Excessive sunbathing can be very bad for the aura, causing it to expand and become very diffuse. You may have noticed a feeling of weakness after prolonged sunbathing and here it is sensible to try to restore the aura to its normal condition by visualizing it very strongly around yourself. Excessive drink has a somewhat similar effect, except that often the etheric body is put completely out of alignment, resulting in an unpleasant feeling of disassociation. Drugs (narcotics) again can severely damage the aura, forcing the mental bodies to 'open out' in an unnatural manner and leaving the physical body unprotected and vulnerable to negative influences, and physical intruders such as germs, viruses, etc. What effect all this would have on the colours of the aura can well be imagined. Sometimes permanent damage results, with a weakness left in the aura which has to be continually patched up. Such weaknesses can also be caused through illness, or some traumatic experience in life, although in these latter cases a good healer may be able to repair the damage.

Dreams

One of the internal manifestations of colour is that experienced in dreams. At least much of the time from those dreams we remember, we have monochrome or black and white dreams, but now and then we will have a dream with outstandingly vivid colouring. This may be due, on the physical level, to chemical or electrical interactions within the brain, or on another level it may be something to do with our innate ability to visualize colour. Whatever the reason, it is again interesting to include symbolic colour along with normal dream interpretation. Jeremy Taylor in his book *Dream Work*[5] puts forward the intriguing idea that people dream in colour most of the time but that mostly women recall colour because they have a general tendency to pay conscious attention to the realms of feeling, 'and to the visual and aesthetic impact of waking life'. He also considers that colour in dreams depends very much on our own emotional life and that this is why red is usually the first colour detected in dream recall — being the colour associated with the most basic and strongest emotions — rage, lust, love, etc.

It seems, according to one scientific experiment[6] that the colours most frequently seen are in the red and orange areas. This would fit in with Jeremy Taylor's point that red is the first colour recalled after black and white. Purples, blues and blue-green were mostly absent. Six male observers were used in this experiment, all of whom had normal colour vision and their dreams were recorded over a period of five months. Immediately after waking they were required to identify on a colour atlas, any colours seen. The experiment does not really seem broad enough in scope or duration to be the final word on dream colour, and other researches reveal a wide discrepancy in the figures quoted. Again, using female subjects may reveal an entirely different pattern of dream colour, as from another survey mentioned in the same article results indicate that 51 per cent of men and only 31 per cent of women never have, or remember, colour dreams, suggesting that dream recall is far greater for women. All that being said, enquiries amongst one's friends and acquaintances usually reveal that someone has had dreams involving colour — and not only red. It may be useful to consider briefly how we can incorporate these colours into our normal dream interpretations. As can be guessed, the colours can be interpreted very much along the lines already described but a brief résumé may be helpful and you can then qualify your interpretation according to the further content of the dream.   •

Red can represent, as said before, passion, anger, strong feelings of various kinds, warmth, life and vitality, depending on other aspects of the dream. Blood and fire are often seen in dreams and the latter is sometimes indicative of a situation likely to get out of control if not carefully watched. Blood is life, and again depending on the content of the dream, can be positive or negative. Red can of course appear in other guises — clothes, hair, sky and so on. As most of us tend to associate red with some kind of danger or excitement it can thus suggest covert desires, or a warning of some kind. You have to use your own common sense here — obviously a cosy little fire would not have the same connotations as a roaring conflagration — the former suggests that a certain situation or project is steadily under way, and the latter that it is likely to get entirely out of hand. The qualities of fire — volatility, instability; but also vitality and potentiality — all add significance to dream material.

Orange is a muted form of red, so one would not allot such strong attributes to it as those of red. Orange is health, enthusiasm and youthfulness and would seem to add a very positive quality to a dream, but here again it must be set against the general tone and feeling of the dream. We associate orange with the sun, with cheerfulness but without the fierce heat of red — a mixture of vitality and wisdom.

Yellow in dreams is another very positive colour, again depending on the dream scenario. It can stand for wisdom, particularly if a dream person appears dressed in yellow or gold — it could represent an inner guide or some wiser aspect of ourselves. Here again common sense must be used in assessing the possibilities of a particular dream. A field of yellow wheat, for example, would appear to show that a very satisfactory outcome of something long planned is coming to fruition and that all is proceeding well; but a yellow desert scene would suggest quite the opposite. However yellow is on the whole a positive colour, indicative of wisdom, clarity and light.

Green in dreams is very much a symbol of life, fertility and creativity. A lush green field of grass, compared with a few tufts in a stony landscape, speaks for itself of at least inner vitality and the possibility of further growth with subsequent harvest. As in other areas of colour interpretation, a murky or disturbed green would suggest an impairment of this happy situation. Generally speaking, green is a positive colour suggesting that one's inner life is full of energy and creativity.

Blue is said to be rarely seen in dreams but this may be just poor recall. It is a quieter colour and maybe not so easy to remember. It represents spirituality, cosmic energy and various emotional levels depending on the content of the dream. In one sense, to see a blue sky or a blue sea could mean that one is simply reproducing an everyday factual scene — or it could mean much more. Blue when associated with water has emotional implications, and as with fire, the difference between a small, still pool and a raging torrent is enormous. In the former case it suggests a need or desire for quiet contemplation; in the latter case it suggests emotions out of control with the dreamer in danger of being swept along by overwhelming feelings. The added coloration of blue will add intensity to such dreams. Blue sky, though, gives a more tranquil, spiritual feeling to a dream, a reaching up, a striving towards the heavens, the qualities of air being lighter, and more exhilarating and detached than those of water. Blue added to an otherwise drab scene could point to a positive and spiritual uplift which would improve an inert phase in one's life. If blue appears in other ways — in clothes, eyes, and so on, care should be taken to set this against the rest of the dream.

Violet and all its subtle variations, is fairly unusual for dreams. It is generally connected with one's inner self, unless of course it is a rather factual dream where you are picking a bunch of violets. Even so, dreams such as these can be interpreted on more levels than one. To dream of purple robes may mean aspirations of power or success, while to dream of amethysts denotes a healing situation. Generally it is a colour connected with spirituality and one's inner life.

Brown in dreams gives a rather dull, negative quality. It can suggest all the earthly qualities of rocks, soil, mud — together with the possibilities of being bogged down, stuck in a rut, or just plodding along — or even a time of aridity, depending on the shade in question. All-brown dreams are fairly uncommon and would perhaps reveal that the dreamer is 'browned-off' with life or going through a dull period.

All-**Grey** dreams emphasize this possibility and indicate a very dreary mental outlook. However, in smaller quantities both these colours have their place in normally coloured dreams.

Black in dreams does not necessarily mean something dire. A black cat crossing one's path points to some good luck coming.

A black human figure can represent the unconscious or sexual side of ourselves. Black animals, depending on the nature of the creature, can be beautiful or menacing; it all depends on the 'feel' of the dream. Black seen in dreams should be set against the other aspects and interpreted accordingly.

White in dreams is not usually seen exclusively, unless it is a snow scene. If you recall such a dream setting it could imply some 'freezing' of the emotions and if everything is completely iced up then you have a bit of a problem! Try melting some of that snow and ice so that little rivers and green fields can appear!

The most rewarding dreams are of course those in several colours. One main colour in an otherwise monochrome dream usually pinpoints a significant aspect, but a whole range of colour suggests balance and harmony. Taken along with a generally positive content this is the most enjoyable kind of dream to have but alas, all too rare for most people.

Meditation
Meditation is a somewhat different activity to that of dreaming, although there are similarities, but the former is usually controlled, the latter only occasionally. While meditating, one can call up a particular colour, either for general contemplation or for a particular purpose, such as healing. Then there are the colours that float through one's mind, or which are associated with the object of meditation. Most meditation teachers instruct one to ignore these passing diversions but it might be worthwhile briefly to note them in passing and later check on their specific meanings, although of course undue importance should not be attached to them.

A meditation on a specific colour is often a useful exercise. It can be generally visualized as either filling the immediate surroundings, or as a cloud in front of one's eyes, or embodied in something symbolic such as a rose, a cup, a pool, a tree and so on. Care should be taken to remember that the object chosen for the colour in question has its own symbolic associations and if you just wish to contemplate pure colour then choose a very simple geometrical shape. Colour cards are a useful prop for this kind of meditation, you can gaze at a particular colour for some moments, and having fixed it in your mind's eye, proceed to visualize it mentally and see what comes.

Another interesting exercise is to take a colour card, without looking to see what colour it is, and place it face down on a table. Then 'tune in' to it and see what comes. This exercise, like any other ESP test, is best done in a small group or with another person. The results can be very illuminating and give you much symbolic imagery to play with afterwards. You may not get the actual colour of the card but you will probably get some sort of sensation with it as described in the earlier section on sightless vision.

A really worthwhile area of experiment is that of mind games. These are not quite meditation in the usual meaning of the word but certainly overlap in some areas. A mind-game is to some extent a 'talk-through' meditation but in another sense it stretches the mind and exercises quite a few dormant faculties. 'Path-working' is another term used for this type of activity but whatever you call it the results can be very beneficial.

You may like to try such a game, incorporating colour visualization as well as using your imagination for the other senses of touch, smell and hearing. With the correct formula and a good 'leader' a group of people can return from such an excursion both refreshed and relaxed. It isn't hypnosis and you are totally in command of your own version of the game. But it is important that the leader takes it fairly slowly, giving people the chance to arrange their inner scenery. A typical example would be as follows. I call it 'Eternity'.

The leader first of all suggests that everyone sits themselves comfortably, relaxed, with feet firmly on the ground and hands gently resting on the knees. A few deep breaths, and/or a body consciousness exercise, will put the participants in the right frame of mind, turning them away from all thoughts of mundane problems. The 'body consciousness' exercise consists of relaxing each part of the body in turn, commencing with the feet, and going on up to the top of the head. This can be combined with closing the aura by visualizing a blue or white light encircling the body, topped with a protective symbol such as a cross or whatever you prefer. This leaves everyone feeling comfortably relaxed and yet protected, and with their train of everyday thoughts broken and dispersed. After a little practice all this only takes a few minutes or so and then the leader can suggest a simple exercise ...

You are walking along the beach on a beautiful sunny day. The sky is an intense blue with a few fluffy white clouds floating around; the sea is sparkling. You can smell the saltiness in the air and feel the crunchiness of the yellow sand beneath your bare feet; hear the swish of the small wavelets as they ebb and flow; feel the golden warmth of the sunshine. In the distance you can see white cliffs, topped with green grass. As you walk along you feel a little breeze brushing your face. After a while you come to a pathway leading away from the beach and up towards the top of the cliff. It is rocky but not too steep and as you climb upwards you pass clumps of pink sea-thrift and brilliant scarlet poppies, growing among the chalky rocks. The path finally leads you out to the top of the cliff. You are up above the sea now, surrounded by lush green grass, daisies and poppies and other flowers. You sit down gratefully, relax, and gaze out to sea. The scintillating stillness of the ocean, reflecting gold and silver lights, and the calm blue of the sky, combine to give you a sense of eternity, timelessness and utter security. You think on this idea for a little while (3-5 minutes) meanwhile enjoying the colours and sensations around you. After this short rest, rise and return back down the rocky path to the beach, all the while continuing to sense the qualities of air, earth, water and fire, and seeing the colours of your surroundings. Once back on the beach, take one last look at the ocean and then let the scene fade from your mind. You are now back in your chair, feeling refreshed and relaxed.

Make sure however, that you are properly 'earthed' by stretching and wriggling about a bit, and by imagining that your aura is still enclosing you. It wouldn't do to remain on Cloud Nine — you might not notice where you were going on the way home, or end up feeling rather disassociated.

This sort of exercise makes a very pleasant end to an evening of discussion, healing, or listening to music. It enlarges your colour visualization capabilities, besides making you more aware of a lot of things you take for granted. An enterprising leader can modify it by introducing further touches such as some little sailing ships with coloured sails; or beach huts in brilliant colours, or can extend the walk to take in a rather more complicated scenario. You can stop to bathe in the sea if you wish, or even have a paddle. For those people who say 'I can't stand heights' or 'I'm frightened of water' the leader must give encouragement and help by explaining that they have complete control over their 'picture' and can modify it, or shut it off, whenever they like. The leader should stress that this type of exercise offers a wonderful opportunity to overcome hang-ups such as these and that by mentally approaching whatever it is that is frightening the sufferer can gradually gain control over it. This sort of exercise is sometimes used in 'aversion therapy' although maybe not with such pleasant spin-offs as 'a nice day at the seaside'.

Yet another exercise can enhance your colour awareness, besides giving you some insights into your own subconscious. This I call 'The Treasure Cave'.

This time, after the usual relaxation procedure, we find ourselves standing outside a cave (those frightened of caves can have a torch or take a gnome with them for company, if they like!). It is an attractive-looking cave, with little green ferns growing around its mouth, and a silver stream trickling down beside it. You enter the cave, which has a faint luminosity of its own so that you can see your way. It is cool inside, and the path is slightly sandy. The sides of the tunnel are smooth and now and again you see the same little green ferns that were growing outside. You walk on along the tunnel, which is gradually descending, lower and lower. (Here give a little time for everyone to make their descent). Eventually the tunnel widens out and you are standing in a vast cave, illuminated by many twinkling points of light. These illuminate the cavern sufficiently to reveal, in front of you, a still, small pool of clear water. You go towards it and sit down beside it, gazing into it. It is not very deep, and has a sandy bottom. Lying on the bottom are many coloured precious stones — amethyst, ruby, pearl, sapphire, emerald, opal, diamond, topaz, together with such semi-precious substances as amber and coral. (You can make this as simple or as complicated as you like.) You are allowed to take *one* of these stones. You put your hand into the water (try to *feel* its wetness and coolness) and take out the stone of your choice. Let us say it is a sapphire. It is a fairly large stone, the size of a walnut. You gaze into its blue depths and it is as if looking into a blue grotto, there is the same sense of timelessness and endurance as we had with the sea, plus the stability and comfort of the earth. You take your stone with you as you rise from beside the pool and retrace your steps back up along the tunnel, again reliving the sensation of coolness, smooth walls, sandy floor. You come out from the cave mouth into soft, warm sunshine to see your chair just outside the cave. Sit in it and come back gently to the present, using the same techniques as before for earthing yourself. You have brought a gift back with you this time — your sapphire. Now you can of course look up any good book of symbology (a couple are suggested at the end of the chapter) and find out for yourself the meaning of a sapphire. But in case you haven't such a reference book to hand, here are a few brief notes on the meanings of such jewels:

Amethyst	—	Humility, peace of mind, sobriety, the stone of healing; bringer of dreams and visions, protection against over-enthusiasm.
Amber	—	Congealed light; courage; gives magic power and protection. Sacred to Apollo and regarded as Freya's tears.
Coral	—	Sea-tree of the Mother-Goddess; longevity, fertility of the waters, ideas, aspiration.
Diamond	—	Light, life, the sun, constancy, innocence, eternity, incorruptability, durability, eternity of spirit.
Emerald	—	Immortality, hope, youth; Spring, growth of spiritual awareness, harmony with life.
Opal	—	Faithfulness, religious intensity, prayers, psychic powers; protection against anger, purification.
Pearl	—	Chastity, purity, the moon, feminine principle, value, beauty that arises from the trials of life.
Ruby	—	Dignity, power, love, passion, beauty, longevity, invulnerability, sympathy, feeling for others.
Sapphire	—	Truth, chastity, spirituality, contemplation and devotion, protection from evil, heavenly attributes.
Topaz	—	Divine goodness, fidelity, friendship, love, sagacity, the sun.

This list should give you some food for thought. Why did you choose such a stone? Was it the colour that attracted you or some other association? Combined with the meanings in the above list and with the colour meanings given earlier, you should be able to compile yourself quite a useful little dossier about why you like a particular colour, thus giving some insight into your inner self. Jewels traditionally symbolize spiritual truths and jewels from a cave refer to the intuitive knowledge hidden in the unconscious.

You may wonder what such exercises have to do with healing — but rest assured, anything that relaxes the body, stimulates the mind, and refreshes the spirit *is* healing. Whatever our state of health, all of us can do with a little healing of one sort or another at times — the stress of everyday modern life, with its vast range of choice and many complications, means we are often tense and anxious without knowing it. A little break now and then will remind us of our priorities.

You may like to try another exercise. I call this 'Belonging'. Begin with the usual relaxation procedure and then imagine you are standing on a beautiful sandy beach in the early hours of the morning, just before the sun is up. All is quiet except for the gentle ripple of wavelets on the shore. You can see the crescent moon high in the sky, and many stars. As you gaze towards the horizon the first faint light of dawn is appearing, a pale pink flush of colour, and the deep blue of the night sky above you becomes paler — a translucent eggshell blue. Slowly the stars all begin to disappear as the dawn light creeps upwards. All except one star, which is the most brilliant. It gives out great flashes of colour, red, green, blue and gold — like a diamond. You contemplate it, knowing that you and it are eternally linked, that you are made of the same star-stuff, forged eons ago and trillions of light years away; composed of the same material as that great star which is now sending huge shafts of light down to you, both of you created in the first great dawn when the universe began.

This star, this cosmic 'relative', has a message for you. It sends out one final great amethyst flash of light as the sky lightens. This amethyst light reaches down to where you are standing and for a moment you and the star are indissolubly linked. Experience the feeling of belonging in the Universe, of being part of it, of knowing you are a child of the stars, and that you have a right to be here as much as that vast sun. You are at one with it as a member of the universe.

Thank the star for its message and, as it finally winks out, turn to look at the sun rising over the horizon. Salute it, as a fellow being, then let the scene fade from your mind and return to your present environment, making sure your aura is 'closed' and you are properly earthed.

The 'message' which this great star sends you may not be an obvious one. It may leave you with an enhanced experience of cosmic consciousness, or something may surface later in your mind, or in a dream. You could try other colours in this exercise and see if you get different results.

Here I suggest a final exercise, in which you can assess how much knowledge you have acquired about colour so far and whether you can use this knowledge in a positive way. It is called 'The Castle'.

Commence with the usual relaxation procedure. Then imagine you are walking on a little path across a meadow towards a white castle in the distance. The day is warm and sunny, the meadow is lush and green, full of wild flowers, chirping crickets and humming bees. There is a peaceful and serene atmosphere. The path is leading you up to the castle, which is fairly large. It has six doorways and over each hangs a beautiful silk flag, each a different colour, scarlet, yellow, soft green, blue, indigo and violet.

Choose one of the doorways and enter the castle. You go up six short steps and enter a hall. This hall is completely coloured in whatever colour flag you chose to go in by — floor, walls, and furniture, and even the light filtering through leaded panes is coloured. You feel completely immersed in this colour, almost as if you are breathing it in. Try to feel its qualities, its warmth or coolness, its stimulation or tranquillity. Feel that the very air around you is coloured. Take what you need from it.

Presently pass through the hall to a door at the far end. Climb another short flight of stairs and this time you enter a hall of pure crystal which reflects back to you many scintillating colours. Here is the heart of your castle. Now take whatever you feel was the best in your colour and place it, in the form of a symbol, on a table in the centre of the hall. The symbol can take any form, a fruit, a flower, an abstract design. Choose it to portray the qualities of your colour choice. This is *your* gift to *your* castle. It lies there secure for you whenever you wish to return. Return through the castle and meadow and finish as before.

A castle represents our inner security; also that which is difficult to attain; it usually holds some treasure. You can use such an exercise to go through the whole colour spectrum. This will help your colour visualization immensely and will fix in your mind the qualities associated with the different colours. It may also give you a pleasant feeling of relaxation and well-being if you are in say a mood that you would like to change. If you feel your mind needs to be stimulated, choose the red or yellow flags; if you need calming, try for blue or green; if you really need to lift your consciousness, try indigo and violet.

What actually comes forth after such mind games and the simple meditation techniques described in this chapter is subject to your own personal interpretation and it is important not to ask someone else to do this for you unless you are really stuck for an answer. The value of the exercise will be lost otherwise. To consider a particular colour may bring scenes and symbols to your mind of a personal nature of which someone else would not know the background. Blue, for instance, may bring memories and associations that may surprise you with their depth. On the other hand they may surprise you with their triviality. But deep or shallow, they are all part of you and worthy of attention. This kind of meditation is fairly low-key but even so can provide valuable insights into one's inner life.

References

1. Exodus 19.30
2. Carlos Castenada *A Separate Reality* (Penguin Books, 1973).
3. Thelma Moss *The Probability of the Impossible* (RKP, 1976).
4. S.G.J.Ouseley, *The Science of the Aura* (L.N.Fowler & Co.Ltd., London, 1949).
5. Jeremy Taylor, *Dream Work* (Fowler Wright Books Ltd., 1983).
6. Charles A. Padgham 'Colours experienced in dreams' *British Journal of Psychology* 66, 1, pp.25-28 (1973)

Further Reading

Harold Saxton Burr, *Blueprint for Immortality* (Neville Spearman, London, 1972).

Carlos Castenada, *The Teachings of Don Juan: a Yaqui Way of Knowledge* (Penguin Books, 1970).

Carlos Castenada, *Journey to Ixtlan* (Penguin Books, 1974).

Walter J. Kilner, *The Human Aura* (University Books, N.Y., 1965).

Max Freedom Long, *The Secret Science Behind Miracles* (Huna Research Publications, Vista, Calif. USA, 1948).

Edward W. Russell, *Design for Destiny* (Neville Spearman, London).

Life Outside the Physical Body, Colour and Reincarnation, The Atlanteans, (1975).

5.
Colour In Our Healing

Colour healing of one type or another has been popular from very early days when colour was first used for symbolic reasons. The ancient Egyptians, Babylonians and Assyrians practised therapeutic sunbathing, and a highly developed sun and airbathing cult existed in ancient Greece and Rome. The old Germanic races likewise regarded the healing power of sunlight very highly and worshipped the rising sun, and the Incas of South America also practised a sun cult called heliotherapy.[1] It is obvious that in these long ago times people were as well aware of the healing value of sunlight as we are today. This may seem to have no direct connection with actual colour healing until we remember that sunlight can be split into the colours of the spectrum and thus contains all of these within itself.

The decision to use individual colours in the form of light rays for specific healing problems must have originated along with the use of plants, flowers, pigments, etc. of a colour corresponding to the disease in question, for example, red flowers etc. being used to treat a blood condition. As this aspect of healing developed, someone along the way had the idea that coloured light might have a similarly efficacious effect.

In the first century AD Aurelius Cornelius Celsus wrote a number of books on medicine which included various coloured ointments and plasters in black, green and white. Claudius Galen, Greek physician to Marcus Aurelius, who was a most celebrated medical writer, mentions colour in his treatises. Then Avicenna, an Arabian philosopher and physician (980-1037) wrote a book, the *Canon of Medicine*. He considered colour most important in diagnosis, relating it to the human temperament and the physical state of the body. For instance, he maintained that to gaze at something red if one were bleeding would make matters worse. In common with Celsus he used coloured flowers in his remedies, matching them by colour to the ailments in question. Then along came a German-Swiss physician and chemist, Theothrastus Bombastus von Hohenheim, who assumed the name of Paracelsus. He held many theories much advanced for his time but didn't have a very good opinion of Galen and Avicenna and publicly burnt their books! Even so, colour was included among the many remedies he used, along with music, herbs, diet, bleeding and purging, and so on.

Since then there have been many practitioners of colour healing of varying degrees of credibility, one of the most outstanding being Edwin D. Babbitt. He was enthusiastically acclaimed by many people but attacked by the medical profession. His book *The Principles of Light and Colour* (1878) created quite a sensation in the field of colour healing. He claimed cures of various ailments by the treatment of sunlight being passed through panes of coloured glass, and invented and sold such aids to colour healing as 'Chromo-Disks', 'Chromo-flasks', a 'Thermolume' cabinet for colour therapy treatment and a type of stained glass window which could also be used for colour healing purposes. He set up a chain of correspondences between colours and the elements and minerals. Babbitt was not quite the first in his field, but he was certainly one of the most spectacular exponents of colour healing. He considered blue and violet to have soothing qualities and therefore regarded them as useful for all inflammatory and nervous conditions, while white and blue were regarded as good for sciatica and rheumatism. You will see later in the chapter that this does not tie in with much present day thinking. Along with many others, he considered red to have a potent effect upon the blood and very helpful in cases of paralysis, while yellow and orange stimulated the nerves. Various arrangements of these colours were used for more complex conditions. His basic principles are however still used today by many colour therapy practitioners, some of whom have developed their own versions of his original work. Naturally the subject remains a matter of controversy and although Babbitt's chromotherapeutic devices and prescriptions are not legally allowed in his country of origin, the United States, in Britain there is a fairly wide choice of colour therapists who use and sell his aids to colour therapy.

Perhaps a few words on cosmic rays will not come amiss at

this point. Many healers talk about working with these 'rays' which may seem puzzling to the uninitiated. These rays are of course those of the light spectrum — the colours of the rainbow. Each ray is regarded as having certain attributes and on the whole these tie in fairly well with colour meanings already outlined. Many healers add to the seven spectrum rays the colours of brown, grey, black and white, sometimes adding an extra shade or two of any one colour. However, in order not to make matters too complicated, we shall only identify eleven of the rays.

When a healer works with a certain colour ray, then he or she intends to utilize all the known positive characteristics of that particular ray and to reinforce this extra ammunition is brought in, in the form of similarly-coloured plants, flowers, vegetables, fruit, colour-charged water, coloured lamps and even coloured clothes. Most deities are associated with one or other of the colour rays and this is where those who engage in ritual of any kind find it important to correlate in colour all the impedimenta used in the ritual. For others, strong visualization of the colour required will be sufficient and while one does not think each time: 'red — that's warmth, life, energy and so on', obviously the person using the rays must have some basic idea of what they represent. To sum up, talk of working with 'cosmic rays' is really just a rather fancy way of saying you are working with certain colour principles. Let us begin with the basics.

Red

This includes every shade and tint from pink to maroon. It is regarded as the ray of Will and Power, life, vitality and energy. It is also symbolic of blood, battles and war and red ray qualities can be found in the symbolism of religious and spiritual movements, signifying the fight against evil. Much talk is made of people being 'on a certain ray' and if you feel you are on a red ray, then you're the pioneering, leader type of person, or would like to be! It is regarded by some healers as a powerful healing agent in diseases of the blood and circulation, general debility and depression. It also inspires heroism and courage.

Orange

This is the ray associated with energy. It has some modified characteristics of the red ray, bringing thought (yellow) to action (red). It therefore brings in qualities of discipline and control to the wilder attributes of red and in some ways has a more practical flavour to it. This colour however should be used carefully as not many people can carry it off well. Nervy people should avoid it. It is thought to be helpful for chest conditions and problems of spleen and kidneys, and for digestive ailments.

Yellow

This is the ray of intellect, mental creativity and a liking for mental employment and activity as opposed to the physical. It is regarded as having a stimulating effect on the nerves, being related to the great glandular centre at the Solar Plexus. Yellow ray people are usually very quick thinkers. At its highest level it is the ray of wisdom although unfortunately it does have some rather dismal connotations. In the main it is a very stimulating ray. It has a powerful effect on the nervous system and is considered suitable for a room where mental pursuits are undertaken. Some healers use this ray for diseases of the skin and nerves.

Green

This is the ray of balance, harmony and sympathy, adaptability and diplomacy. Used wisely, it should ideally sort out different levels of a situation so that a suitable compromise is reached. It can be a good tonic for tired 'nerves' and its changeable quality also helps prevent stagnation. There is however the danger that green-ray persons may find themselves sitting on both sides of the fence at once! Green being a mixture of blue-yellow (love-wisdom) it is said to influence the heart centre, healing and soothing emotional disorders and nervous headaches. It is to a great extent the colour of our planet and to gaze at green fields, trees and plants has a very soothing effect. Even so, for the highly nervous it may not have such a beneficial result, as in the case of someone who was unhappy living in the country and who really required a more stimulating environment. Sometimes the force of nature can be really overwhelming to people who are not in a good state of balance and as such, although it is a ray of inexhaustible energy, it must be used with care.

Blue

Blue is usually regarded as the 'love' ray on its highest plane. It symbolizes harmony, truth, serenity and helps raise the consciousness to a spiritual level. It soothes and calms the mind, but can be rather cool and thus can be used for cleansing, for fighting feverish conditions, bleeding, and nervous irritations. All the previously mentioned characteristics of blue come together in this ray, which is only superseded by its higher counterpart, **Indigo**, which is the ray of spirituality, devotion, intuition and dedication. It holds a hint of mystery and can at times be cold and dispassionate but a true indigo, like the evening sky, suggests inner light of a quality to offset cooler attributes. It is astringent, purifying and said to influence the organs of sight, hearing and smelling and thus used for diseases of the eye, ear and nose.

Amethyst
This is the ray connected with ceremony, ritual and magic but also that of spiritual and mental equilibrium. It is a useful ray for tranquillizing a troubled situation. This ray influences the highest in man and can be spiritually healing and purifying, aiding sleep, and the development of psychic abilities. Those rare folk on a true amethyst ray are the peacemakers in the world.

Purple and Violet follow on, with more of red (will and power) accompanying the qualities of spirituality and calmness, so it is not surprising that it is used so much for ritual, both secular and religious. On its lower levels it can indicate pride and pomposity but on to the violet end it is considered to be equivalent to the highest and most evolved state of consciousness. No wonder, as you will see later, it helps 'repel nasty spirits'! Violet is used by some for the treatment of mental and nervous problems, neuralgia, rheumatism and epilepsy.

Brown
This is similar to green in that it is a ray of balance but has to be used with discretion. The term 'brown study' aptly describes its qualities of concentration and acquisition of knowledge. It can be rather heavy but small quantities are essential to 'earth' a situation or personality that has become rather out of hand.

Grey
At its highest silvery hue grey is the ray of peace; darker shades indicate persistence and spiritual struggle. There are some

people who seem to be 'silver-ray' persons — if of the silvery hue, there seems something mercurial, light and elusive about them; on the darker level they are just as difficult to get through to, but of a denser vibration.

Black

While obviously not used in orthodox healing, it still has a place amongst the other rays. Its purpose is to absorb and store away secretly — much as the colour black absorbs all other colours, giving none out. Its restrictive and protective qualities are useful for those who wish to keep their mysteries hidden from the gaze of the uninitiated. Perhaps if you are on this ray you are an aspiring magician of a very secret order!

The above is of course a very simplified list of the meanings attributed to the colour rays. And it does not mean that because you like a certain colour that you are 'on' that ray! It takes honest self-examination and maybe an even more honest friend before one can really be considered as 'on a certain ray'. In fact most of us are a mixture of rays, in this sense, with perhaps one more predominant than the others. Suggestions for those who wish to study the subject more in depth are given at the end of the chapter.

It is hoped that this will give some idea of how 'cosmic rays' are used. For healing, these rays can be applied for their qualities on all levels — mental, physical and spiritual.

Practical aids

One of the most well-known colour therapists in Britain is Theo Gimbel, who runs the Hygeia Clinic in Gloucester. He has also published a number of books on the subject of colour healing and has some very interesting things to say on the subject. His father, Max Gümbel-Seiling, worked with Rudolf Steiner between 1912 and 1925. They evolved a system of colours for stage lighting and practical use whereby appropriate colours can be made to suggest certain atmospheres, for example, a rainbow for spirituality; black and grey for a sombre or macabre situation; red for joyful activity; blue for sympathy, devotion, and so on. White suggests angels and brides, while black is reminiscent of a priest, a judge — or the devil! Grey reminds us of ghosts, dusk and dawn and all in-between states; violet — magic and mystical states; brown — down to earth and matter-of-fact things. The Anthroposophical Society, of which Rudolf Steiner was the founder, have of course done an immense amount of work on various types of colour therapy, particularly in the field of artistic expression. Theo Gimbel has obviously been much influenced by their work and that of Babbitt to some extent, but has clearly expanded on both these methods and evolved a comprehensive system of his own. He maintains for instance, that children up to the age of three or so see colours in their complementaries — if looking at green the child will see magenta. He considers therefore that pregnant women should wear white, orange or red as these colours do not interfere with the natural (reversed) perception of the embryo. As an embryo, accordingly, the only colour we experience is a deep blue. This ties in somewhat with Dr Buck's theories of the evolution of the colour sense. It might also explain why blue is such a significant colour inasmuch as one wishes to 'sink into it' if one is feeling stressed; it might be a desire to 'return to the womb'.

Gimbel also assigns various colours to different areas of the spine, giving corresponding link-ups with music and astrology. He considers the connection between the spine and the sound of the whole human skeleton to be most significant. Amongst the aids to therapy which he uses are 16 different filters which form part of the treatment in his colour therapy room. This is generally bathed in a blue light which is filtered through variously shaped apertures onto whichever part of the body needs healing. His books give clear instructions as to how to proceed with colour therapy on a purely mental basis but it would undoubtedly prove more valuable to undergo a training period at his clinic. This system of colour filters for chromotherapy is quite popular, most healers using a lamp or projector into which the filters can be inserted, or the patient can sit in a Dr Babbitt-type 'Thermolume' cabinet and be bathed in colour from various screens fixed at the front of it.

Another method widely used is that of wrapping a colour filter around a glass of water and placing it in the sunlight for an hour or so. The water is then drunk or used for bathing any afflicted areas. This is one of the methods favoured by the College of Psychotherapeutics, White Lodge, Spalding, Kent, where it is also possible to stay for the purposes of treatment and/or study.

A variation on the above methods is that used at the Château de Caulet Relaxarium at Mazerolles-du-Razes in France, where patients can lie and sunbathe comfortably under colour filter screens. These treatments are co-ordinated with yoga and other therapeutic exercises in peaceful country surroundings.

A further system combining colour therapy and yoga is outlined by Annie Wilson and Lilla Bek in their book *What Colour Are You?*[2] The authors work on the chakric centres of the body through various yoga exercises. Detailed instructions and photographs outline this system of therapy. I do however strongly feel that yoga needs to be personally taught, otherwise one may adopt an incorrect position which may be very difficult to eradicate and which may do more harm than good.

Chakric healing

Many colour healers work on the chakric points. The chakras are places in the auric body where energy is centralized, as it were. Usually regarded as seven in number, they are seen clairvoyantly as whirling vortices of light. If well balanced and working properly, then it's 'all systems go'. But if not it is assumed that a rebalancing treatment is necessary. The chakras tend to influence that part of the physical body in which they are situated and their colours and attributes correspond to the rainbow spectrum, as follows, so it is easy enough to remember them.

Location	Colour	Attribute
Crown of head/pituitary	Violet	Spirituality/philosophy
Forehead (third eye)/ pineal	Blue	Clairvoyance
Throat-Thyroid	Turquoise	Intelligence/ Clairaudience
Heart	Green	Understanding/ Compassion
Stomach/solar plexus	Yellow	Feeling
Adrenals/side kidneys	Orange	Feeling/Sensation
Sacral/base of spine	Red	Sexual energy/ Procreation

Healing to the chakra in question is usually given in the form of colour replenishment. The chakras are however usually in a very delicate state of balance and inexperienced healers should *not* attempt to interfere with them or they could make matters worse. Many healers combine yoga and massage with chakric colour therapy.

Mary Anderson, in her excellent book *Colour Healing*[3] recommends colour breathing, which she considers as important as the drinking of colour-charged water. One is shown by means of instructions in the book, how to breathe in the required colour. Again the chakras are an important link with the colour therapy but the author does advise that a colour therapist be consulted. Generally the treatments follow the line of colour correspondences, as with red fruit and vegetables being combined with red-charged water for conditions such as anaemia, with further treatment of red light applied to the soles of the feet and to the 'red' chakra at the base of the spine. Many other illustrations are given for treatment along the lines described. The author goes on to describe briefly a system of gem therapy practised in India. The gems are set in a rotating disc in such a way that their rays will fall on a patient's photograph. This method does not fall into the usual colour correspondence system apart from the ruby, which is considered to resonate to the red cosmic ray and the sun and is therefore used for treating heart diseases, anaemia and similar complaints. Dr Bhattacharyya, the exponent of this particular system, considers Pearl — the moon, to reflect the orange cosmic ray; coral — Mars, the yellow cosmic ray, and so on. He has two interesting big guns which he brings in however — the Onyx, which is said to carry the ultraviolet frequency, and the Cat's Eye, which carries the infra-red.

Ms Anderson also outlines a further system of working with colours, numbers and music, with correspondences in fruit and vegetables depending on the particular cosmic ray used.

Perfume can also be combined with colour and music for healing purposes and such a method is described in Roland Hunt's *Fragrant and Radiant Healing Symphony*.[4] Again, the author works with cosmic rays and their correspondences in perfume, music and coloured lamps.

Then there is a method of healing by crystals, which can either be charged with pure white light or with whatever colour is required. This is available from the Crystal Healing Centre[5] at Sherborne, Dorset, and this type of healing is again used to correct chakric imbalances and is frequently combined with yoga, massage and various other alternative remedies. Possibly, in this instance, crystals afford some measure of amplification for the healing energies.

It is possible to try a few experiments for yourself with coloured lights to see how they affect your mood and general well-being. Try red or orange and to a lesser extent yellow generally to raise body temperature and to cheer yourself up or stimulate your mind. You will probably find a short time in such drastic lighting is quite enough. Bright green or blue light will slow the heartbeat and lower body temperature but it may not be advisable to switch from one or the other too suddenly! Many shops nowadays give one the opportunity to experience at first hand such sudden changes of 'atmosphere', so it is not at all necessary to put oneself to the expense of buying specially coloured lamps when one can try out these sensations for free!

'Mind Power' colour healing

From these rather practical aids to colour therapy we come to the healers who use colour in a more subjective sense — that of visualizing and sending colour either in direct or absent healing. Many healers use this method and have their own interpretations of colour by which they work. However I am only going to describe one such method in detail here, which is that used by the Atlanteans.

The Atlanteans is a philosophical organisation which has interests in all New Age subjects including meditation, self-awareness, ESP, the Nature Kingdoms, and of course Atlantis! However, one of its primary functions is that of healing, self-healing as well as that used for other people. Before we dip too deeply into their healing methods, we shall consider a few other opinions. We have seen how in the past colour awareness has developed, particularly in regard to healing, and we can see how the various correspondences have built up between ailments and the plants, fruits, etc. used to cure them. This still applies in colour healing by mind power, although each healer tends to make an individual interpretation.

Most healers tend to agree that **blue** is a healing, cleansing, calming colour. **White** is also often used for general healing. This is the point where healers tend to part company, for use of colours beyond these two is widely individual. As an Atlantean healer, I might be horrified at the idea of sending **red** to anyone except for a specific purpose, such as described later. But some healers find it very useful for treating depression, anaemia and similar conditions. Again, **yellow** is a fairly controversial colour (I am not here equating it with the sun or 'golden light') but according to one school of thought it stimulates mental powers and circulates energy. **Green**, a colour to be used with some caution as it can be rather depressive, is suggested as good for 'expectant mothers and homosexuals'![6] And it may well be, as used by this particular school of thought. It only goes to show how widely divergent are the opinions of colour therapists. Some suggestions are rather simplistic, such as purple — being a colour with religious connotations — repelling nasty spirits! As a first line of defence however it is very useful. Many healers recommend surrounding a patient with 'light' which of course includes all colours. This is an excellent suggestion but for those who wish to be a little more specific a course of colour healing would be the best way of getting off on the right foot. Colour healing can be quite complex and if you start off with a hit and miss attitude, you probably won't do much harm, but you won't do much good either. It is far better to get some initial practical training at first hand. As you become more experienced you can begin to develop your own style. Most healers seem agreed however that red and green must be used very carefully; blue and turquoise are about the most helpful for relaxing the body and cleansing; and yellow and orange, while revitalizing, have again to be used sparingly.

The Atlanteans take the view that for specific healing cases it is necessary to work with at least one or two other persons and that to begin with at least one of the group should have had some personal tuition. However good correspondence courses are there is nothing like being shown how to do something and being able to ask questions and compare notes. Unfortunately there are many people who would love to do this and who have a great desire to help in the world, but who are unable, for reasons of location, work or domestic difficulties, to join a group or take part in residential courses. The Atlanteans have produced a course for such people[7] which, while it does not include the detailed instruction given to healers in a group, is sufficiently structured so as to give a frame of reference from which to begin. Six simple lessons give basic instruction in care of the aura, concentration, meditation, visualization, and techniques of prayer and absent healing, designed in a way to protect the student and to concentrate the healing powers not only on others, but on oneself.

It might appear from this course that too great an emphasis is laid upon protection of healer and patient and many people ask,

'What is there to be afraid of?' and, 'if healing is sent with love, what can cause harm'. All very nice sentiments but a little unrealistic. The best of intentions does not guarantee you immunity from either physical or mental 'invaders' and it is only sensible to take reasonable precautions. Very few of us are adepts, able to walk through the world and by the power of our thoughts pass unharmed through all kinds of dangers. Would you wander around a slum area known for its muggings and violence, without some form of defence, unless you had to? Do you leave your front door or car door unlocked? Love alone won't keep burglars at bay, you have to take precautions on all levels, lock the door on the physical level, put a strong thought, prayer or whatever for the protection of the property on a mental level and finally, if you wish, leave a thought of love for whoever is so out of balance with themselves as to want to injure someone's else's property, thus completing the three levels of physical, mental and spiritual. Of course, we all take chances, hoping it won't happen to us. I for one certainly do not always remember, after locking the door, either of the other two precautions! (For those who wish to investigate these ideas in greater depth I suggest reading Murry Hope's new book *Practical Techniques of Psychic Self Defence*. Ms Hope is one of the founder members of the Atlanteans and as such has these techniques at her fingertips.)[8]

But with healing, it is very important that you be protected on all three levels and it is wiser not to 'take chances'. In my early days of healing I heard of a number of cases where well-meaning unexperienced healers had tried to help someone by 'drawing off' a malignant illness. In one instance at least, which we heard of, the patient recovered and the healer got the disease instead. Regularly in one psychic magazine can be seen anxious queries as to what can be done to throw off a condition picked up from a patient. In a recent issue[9] a reader states that after doing healing on a friend 'I had great difficulty in breathing and realised that the person healed had suffered from a chest complaint.' If the healer is experienced this can probably be thrown off without too much difficulty but if the healer is inexperienced then it may prove much more difficult. Isn't it easier to take precautions to begin with? These are of course extreme cases, but it can happen.

There is no fear motivation behind the teaching of protective measures in Atlantean healing, simply sensible precautions.

Healers can pass things on to patients sometimes that the patients may not want, and although most people unconsciously reject any unwanted transmissions of any nature, an ailing or seriously ill person would not have a strong defence mechanism and might be unable to resist.

Atlantean healing technique
The most basic level on which to prepare yourself for healing is, naturally, the physical one. To be in a comfortable position, relaxed but alert, not hungry but not having just eaten a heavy meal, will set the scene for maybe the most important aspect of Atlantean healing — the control of the aura. The course describes in some detail the functions of the aura and how to keep it in good trim. To start with one undertakes a 'body consciousness' exercise which entails beginning at the feet and slowly working upwards, becoming aware of and relaxing each part of the body in turn, until the top of the head is reached. If your mind happens to wander during this exercise then I am afraid you have to start again from the feet. After this has been successfully completed, you can do the exercise again, this time drawing up around yourself blue or white light until you are completely cocooned in it. If you find this difficult you can imagine stepping into a blue plastic bag, drawing it up around yourself and sealing it at the top with a cross, or ankh, or whatever symbol you would normally use for protection. It is however extremely important that you be as relaxed as possible and if you complete the body consciousness exercise correctly, you should be feeling very relaxed. You can also take a few deep breaths as well. This technique is used for patients as well as healers working on their own, as a patient receiving direct healing who is in an unrelaxed state is not likely to receive much benefit from the healing.

Of course the aura is an emanation from the spirit and as such is always radiating out from the body, but the above exercise will reinforce and strengthen it. Be aware that your mind can control it, you could try a few auric colour changes and check with a fellow healer as to what colour they can see. You can blow your aura out or completely withdraw it so that it cannot be seen, but whatever you do, don't forget it! *Always* do your healing through the filter of your aura — you can imagine it as a very fine mesh which only lets through the highest cosmic energies. If you suspect it has been damaged, either do the body consciousness exercise on yourself, strongly visualizing that the affected part is being repaired, or get another healer to do so. Even a small cut causes the aura to break, and should be repaired immediately. This you can do for yourself by drawing on the cosmic energies, imagining them coming down *through your aura* and through the top of your head and down and out through your fingertips. Hold your hands for a couple of minutes (it seems quite a long time) over the site of the injury and imagine the energy repairing the tear in the aura, a bit like darning a sock! Perhaps the following example will give you some idea of how it works.

A friend of mine, who besides being an Atlantean healer, has also been a nurse, was one day talking (during a tea break, of course) to the Works Sister at her place of employment. They had previously discussed healing and my friend had been explaining that Atlantean healing mostly means work on the aura. 'Is the aura that light I can see around everyone' suddenly asked Sister, 'and why does it have a break in it if someone hurts themselves?' She said she had seen this 'light' around people for many years but did not know what it meant. My friend explained, and mentioned healing the aura, as described above. 'Oh, just a minute then' said the Sister, popping out of the room. She came back with a cut on her finger which was bleeding. 'Can you heal that?' she asked. My friend began visualizing energy streaming from her hands. She held them above the cut finger, sealing off the small cut in the aura. 'I can see a blue light coming from your hands' said Sister, 'the bleeding has stopped too.' Unfortunately this lady became rather frightened about her ability to see the aura and thereafter tended to avoid the subject. Perhaps one day she will be able to look at the whole subject in an objective manner.

This is a fairly simple illustration of how a break in the aura can be sealed — and also how someone can see the aura without actually knowing it! For cases of extreme shock, general injury, as compared with minor problems, one would need to be able to visualize the whole of the aura, re-align it with the body, and seal it carefully. This would best be done by an experienced healer or group of healers. This technique is however very useful for lesser bumps, bruises and burns. Speaking from experience I know it to be very effective, often preventing a bruise or burn if caught in time. Blue or white light can be used, although of course some healers use a colourless ray. It all depends how you feel about a particular case.

White therefore covers a broad area in Atlantean healing. It can be used to recharge and seal the aura, for yourself or someone else. In fact most simple physical problems can be dealt with by white or blue. Sometimes there is a necessity for a soothing, gentle colour for relief of pain and tension. Here we use **coral** and **pink** with its suggestion of warmth and comfort. But it sometimes takes a bit of practice to achieve this colour, whereas red is easier to visualize but you certainly wouldn't use that for soothing. **Red** in fact is rarely used in Atlantean healing, being reserved for certain ulcerous conditions which need drying up, and never for any type of mental healing.

Lilac is occasionally used but it is rather 'heavy' and needs a good build-up of power to achieve any potency. It is therefore best left to experienced healers. Its function is to replenish and rebuild.

Green, as mentioned before, is only used sparingly. It can be used to calm the over-active or even violent person but it is not considered suitable for people suffering from nervous tension or cases of depression, as it may create even more negativity.

Yellow is a colour not normally used, or perhaps only in very special circumstances. It is very mentally stimulating and thought to have a temporary brightening effect which then, if overdone, can produce exhaustion and subsequent depress.

So normally Atlantean healers use only three basic colours — white, blue and coral. Silver and gold are sometimes used in mental healing (for psychological cases) or for conditions associated with the head and eyes.

Many healers prefer not to use colour although often, as in the case of the cut finger mentioned previously, a clairvoyant will see a colour (in this instance blue) when the healer has not been consciously visualizing it.

Earlier exercises in colour visualization will help to concentrate the mind to a point where these colours can be used. But for the purposes of the Atlantean course for 'lone healers' it is not necessary. In any case if one finds it difficult to visualize colour, as many people do, just think of the sensation you wish to transmit — hot, cold, soothing, stimulating, cleansing and so on. But most beginners find it easy to visualize white and blue and once experience is gained, colours can either be abandoned or evolved further depending on the direction one's healing abilities take.

There are many other colour healers and therapists working along these lines and it is not possible to mention them all. Healing comes in many guises and one has to shop around a bit to find one's own particular wavelength. What may suit one person may not suit another and physical problems of a severe nature may need treatment of an orthodox medical nature. If however this can be combined with 'healing' of some kind, it then means that the whole person is being treated on all levels rather than for an isolated and localized medical condition. For those not actually ill there are still the problems of tiredness, stress, worry and so on, which prevent one from enjoying life and exploring one's potential to the full. This is where alternative methods of healing tend to come into their own, providing a wide range of treatments. This is not to discount, of course, the fact that alternative healing methods do produce positive cures for all sorts of conditions and often in cases where normal medical treatment has failed. It all depends, as said before, on one finding the right 'wavelength'.

Colour is an indispensable factor in our lives — let us be more aware of it, enjoy it, and exploit it to the full — and even if perhaps we can't see some colours all that well we can still become conscious of their potency in some of the ways outlined in this book. Let's try and make ourselves a more colour-full, cheerful and exciting new world!

References

1. F. Ellinger as mentioned in *Color and Human Response*, Faber Birren (Van Nostrand Reinhold Co.Inc. USA, 1978).
2. Annie Wilson & Lilla Bek, *What Colour Are You?* (Turnstone Press Ltd., 1982).
3. Mary Anderson, *Colour Healing* (The Aquarian Press, 1979).
4. Roland Hunt, *Fragrant and Radiant Healing Symphony* (H.G.White 1949).
5. Crystal Healing Centre, J. & J. Harvey, Middle Piccadilly, Holwell, Sherborne, Dorset. Tel. Bishops Caundle 468.

6. Francoise Strachan, *Natural Magic* (Marshall Cavendish Publications Ltd., 1974).
7. *Healing in the World Today* (Atlanteans Association Ltd., 1977). An Atlantean Study Course including basic instructions on how to heal. Obtainable from the Atlanteans, Runnings Park, Croft Bank, West Malvern, Worcs. price £1.75.
8. Murry Hope, *Practical Techniques of Psychic Self Defence* (The Aquarian Press, 1983).
9. *Prediction*, December 1983.

Further Reading

Theo Gimbel, *Healing Through Colour* (The C.W. Daniel Co.Ltd., 1980).
Theo Gimbel, *Key, Lock and Door* (Hygeia Publications 1976).
S.G.J. Ouseley, *Colour Meditations* (L.N. Fowler & Co.Ltd., 1949).
James Sturzaker, *The Twelve Rays* (The Aquarian Press, 1976).

Index